Complex Social Issues and the Perinatal Woman

Laura Abbott
Editor

Complex Social Issues and the Perinatal Woman

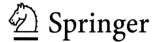 Springer

Editor
Laura Abbott
Department of Allied Health and Midwifery
University of Hertfordshire
Hatfield
Hertfordshire
UK

ISBN 978-3-030-58084-1   ISBN 978-3-030-58085-8   (eBook)
https://doi.org/10.1007/978-3-030-58085-8

This Springer imprint is published by the registered company Springer Nature Switzerland AG
The registered company address is: Gewerbestrasse 11, 6330 Cham, Switzerland

Contents

Introduction

Laura Abbott

This book has evolved through a recognition that a considerable proportion of perinatal women face multidimensional complexities. Health care professionals have a duty to be knowledgeable of those needs, acting with professionalism and compassion. The latest Mothers and Babies: Reducing Risk through Audits and Confidential Enquiries across the UK (MBRRACE-UK) [1] clearly demonstrates the consequences that having multiple complexities has and the need to ensure that susceptible groups receive tailored, timely care. There are substantial changes to maternity services in the United Kingdom (UK) proposed over the next ten years, through the maternity transformation programme, via the National Health Service (NHS) Long Term plan. Meeting the needs of all women is essential to attaining excellence in the twenty-first century care provision as outlined by the National Institute for Health and Care Excellence (NICE) [2, 3]. There is also a need for a concentrated and sustained focus on the findings from MBRRACE-UK. Maternal mortality and stillbirth rates are increasing for women who are from Black, Asian and Minority ethnicities and for women experiencing extreme disadvantage and the need to work together with women to address the shortcomings of maternity services is urgent.

Our book aims to seek to increase our knowledge of some of the complexities facing women and their families. The chapters are written by experts in their field from a variety of backgrounds. Some are experts through experience, and others have significant third sector expertise bringing together their skills of peer care provision and an understanding of the unique needs of the women and families they support. It is the first piece of work to bring together a blend of health care professionals, people with lived experiences and charity workers with expertise in caring for and supporting perinatal women with complex social issues. Pursuing a multidisciplinary approach, this book demonstrates the best quality care for pregnant women and new mothers who may have complex social needs.

The book hopes to amplify voices by highlighting experiences; these are in turn combined with recommendations from specialists in the field, offering a unique mix of compassion and evidence-based guidance. From substance abuse, domestic violence and HIV to experiences of Black, Asian and Ethnic Minorities, homelessness and women in prison, it addresses a range of social issues and provides essential information on how they can best be met. This book will benefit all health and social care professionals working in women's health, whilst also providing a valuable reference guide for maternity departments. We also look at how using a trauma-informed approach can be applied universally to care for all women and hear from charities such as Birth Companions, the 4M project and the Salamander Trust, and how different approaches may directly impact women's care.

This book serves as a guide to understand more with greater compassion and empathy and suggests the adoption of the universal precaution of trauma-informed care approaches. At the heart of the care we give women should be kindness but also continuity in order that we get to know her—working in partnership. The NHS long-term plan and Better Births [4] is timely in ensuring that we provide seamless, high-quality continuity of care to all women when we understand the outcomes are reduced morbidity, mortality and perinatal mental ill health. It is therefore important to understand the impact that delivering the high standards of care required can have on the caregiver. Burnout can be high amongst those who care deeply, and we also need to recognise that.

Each chapter details issues affecting women, often through lives interwoven with abuse, violence and poverty impacting their children. The aim is not to depict women as victims of their circumstances, rather to find ways to deliver multi-agency continuity of care, being aware of our bias and professional responsibilities and understanding how we can and must take a holistic approach. A common thread throughout and one detailed in **Naomi Delap's** chapter is how using a trauma-informed approach provides best practice. A shared problem for many women facing complex social issues is a past experience of trauma. Delap who is the Director of the charity Birth Companions suggests that:

> women whose lives have been shaped by trauma can be particularly vulnerable to its impact during the perinatal period…experiences of trauma have been established as a risk factor for a range of vulnerabilities and poor outcomes during the perinatal period including perinatal depression, PTSD, poor obstetric outcomes and problematic attachment.

Delap's chapter discusses the adverse effect of childhood and adult experiences of trauma and how multiple and gendered experiences of trauma can amplify its impact. It explores the effects of trauma on women during pregnancy, birth and the postpartum period; examines existing trauma-related practice in maternal health and looks at the case for the introduction of a trauma-informed approach within maternity services.

Jennifer Parker, a registered midwife, examines perinatal mental health, its impact, stigma, current midwifery practices and education, through the lens of a woman experiencing in vitro fertilisation (IVF). Looking at the current research and literature, Parker explores the effects of poor perinatal mental health and current practices. Midwifery education in perinatal mental health is scarce, and Parker suggests that improvements could lead to reduced stigma, better detection and consequently more women receiving treatment. At least 80,000 women a year in the UK suffer with generalised anxiety disorder, but the vast majority are either without effective treatment or in most circumstances undiagnosed; this can lead to significant detriments to both the women and their babies? health.

Suzanne Reynolds, a specialist midwife, guides the reader in understanding the statutory instruments for perinatal women experiencing homelessness—an example being that women who are in the third trimester of pregnancy are given 'notice to quit' from hostels. Whilst considered a priority need by local authorities—this makes the homeless woman less visible to professionals who need to find creative ways of engaging with women. Drawing on Reynolds primary research with pregnant women who experience homelessness demonstrates current experiences such as physical health issues, toxic stress [5], mental strain all increasing a woman's morbidity. Continuity of care can be difficult due to the transient nature of homelessness, yet the expert care benchmarked by Reynold's specialist role as midwife for homeless perinatal women is recommended in areas where homelessness is widespread.

Undeniably, homelessness may be a situation often preceded from other complex challenges for a woman—she may be seeking asylum, have experienced domestic abuse or may have been involved in the criminal justice system. **Carolyn Hill's** expertise as a Registered Nurse and Senior Lecturer draws us into a greater understanding of the global issues facing asylum seekers and refugees and whilst defining refugee and migrant status, alerts us to how women may access health care (or not) and how they may have experienced violence and be survivors of trauma. Hill's chapter outlines some of the many issues that the perinatal woman, seeking refuge, may encounter. It begins with the process of seeking asylum and the difficulties associated with providing evidence of being an asylum seeker. There is a brief focus on housing, benefits and access to health care, highlighting the misconceptions held by many in the host country, that asylum seekers and refugees jump to the head of the housing queue, receive better financial support than others already living in the UK and are only in the country to make use of the National Health Service. Matters focusing around the violence some women may have suffered and their physical health are discussed together with issues of psychological trauma.

Principal Lecturer in Social work, **Karen Mill's** draws upon lessons from serious case reviews providing a deeper understanding that drug misuse does not occur in a silo but rather coincides with issues such as poverty, homelessness and involvement with child protection services. MMBRACE-UK [6] outlines how women who misuse drugs and alcohol may book late for antenatal care or miss appointments and Mill's guides the reader in how we can better engage with women, increasing our awareness to the emotional responses such as guilt, balancing risk-taking behaviours and being 'over-optimistic' whilst considering child protection. Importantly, Mill's suggests that the perinatal period may be a catalyst for change in the woman, and therefore tailored antenatal services are indeed vital.

Tawanda Bvumburai, a Complex Social Care and FGM specialist midwife, explores Black Asian Minority Ethnic (BAME) Women's Experiences of Maternity Care in the context of the history and evolution of racism in her chapter. MMBRACE (2020) is a stark reminder that women and babies who are Black, Asian and/or from minority ethnic communities (BAME) are more likely to die than white women. Bvumburai inspires the reader to be honest about why this might be the case and consider all women in minorities. With a mortality rate five times higher than their white counterparts and babies more likely to die, Bvumburai shines a light on the experiences of Black, Asian and Minority Ethnic women and maternity staff. Drawing upon an audit of experiences of women from Black, Asian and Minority ethnicities, Bvumburai encourages the reader to challenge their own prejudice and reflect upon how we should be addressing any bias with the urgency that the latest MBRRACE report calls for.

Celia Wildeman, a senior lecturer in midwifery and counsellor with expertise in family violence, describes an increase in 'domestic' violence experienced by women, suggesting that much of this is still hidden, especially from health care professionals. Domestic violence and abuse have a catastrophic effect on society and affects women from physical, social, psychological and financial perspectives. Evidence suggests that violence can be initiated or escalated in pregnancy and this has serious consequences for the safety of women and babies and care provision. She compels us to examine barriers to care drawing upon her research, with midwives having a significant role in ensuring that lasting and meaningful change occur.

Laura Abbott, a senior lecturer in midwifery and qualitative researcher, explores the human rights and health needs for perinatal women in prison and makes recommendations for best practice and care. Drawing upon her qualitative research, the reader is invited to consider the experiences pregnant women in prison may face. Abbott's chapter deliberates the demographics and characteristics of women in prison who are often from backgrounds of extreme and multiple disadvantage. The health outcomes are explored alongside the psychological impact of imprisonment. One conclusion of the research is that pregnant prisoners are a misfit in the prison system, and they subsequently experience shame and do not always get what they are entitled to. Throughout the chapter, the reader is asked to reflect upon their professional responsibilities and to examine pre-conceived ideas when caring for the pregnant prisoner.

The authors **Angelina Namiba, Longret Kwardem, Rebecca Mbewe, Fungai Murau, Susan Bewley, Shema Tariq and Alice Welbourn** write from their experiences of leading, facilitating and being perinatal peer mentors with, and for women living with an HIV diagnosis in the UK. They support us to consider the experiences of women with HIV and how they may have significant unmet needs especially in relation to poverty, violence and housing. Addressing the stigma and stereotypes affecting women, they explore how peer support, particularly *'mentor mothers'* can support and empower women with HIV status dispelling myths:

> *It was an opportunity to process the past, open very guarded doors, get angry, and be with my pain. Time is so precious, and time to belong, to experience empathy and support, to feel a sense of togetherness allowed me to become strong, in a more powerful way than resilience.* (Mentor Mother)

Through the 4M project (*my health, my choice, my child, my life*) Namiba et al. explore the personal and professional growth of women living with HIV and provide health care professionals with essential guidelines for care.

Paulina Sporek de Lacerda, a registered midwife, Maternity Improvement Advisor and founder of the charity *Deafnest*, explores disability in her chapter about deaf parents. Sporek de Lacerda describes the considerable obstacles that deaf parents may face, despite knowing that little has been done in relation to pregnancy and childbirth. The links between the social exclusion, vulnerability and adverse pregnancy outcomes are well known. Consequently, there is an acute need to train midwives and other medical staff in deaf awareness and associated communication skills. The fact that being deaf is viewed negatively in our society creates complicated interactions between deaf parents and the hearing professionals with whom they come in contact. Sporek de Lacerda discusses the barriers deaf families encounter, including discriminatory health and social support services and limited access to information. Additionally, Sporek de Lacerda suggests that the lack of relevant literature suggests that deafness and pregnancy are two concepts rarely considered together.

Abbi Ayers, the senior coordinator for prison services and breastfeeding lead at the charity Birth Companions, exposes the barriers and contextualises the potential for breastfeeding to trigger past trauma, especially for survivors of sexual abuse. Ayers invites us to consider the differences in ages of babies when breastfeeding and the potential for re-traumatising whilst also describing how survivors may also be empowered. Ayers discusses how breastfeeding support can be an ambiguous definition, prone to interpretation on several levels. For example, direct breastfeeding support may entail intensive one-to-one contact between a caregiver and a postnatal mother, whereas indirect breastfeeding support might include fostering a positive breastfeeding culture or facilitating regular opportunities for expectant mothers to ask questions and access information about their infant feeding choices. For the most part, all women need some form of direct and indirect breastfeeding support if they are to be able to successfully initiate and establish breastfeeding. Ayer's extensive experience of offering breastfeeding support to women who have complex needs has led to the suggestion to take a step back from conventional and generic support models to be able to consider things from a different perspective. The women not only need evidence-based information and practical support with breastfeeding, they also need trauma-informed care, specialist advice and guidance, and non-judgmental acceptance and empathy as they make the infant feeding choices that are right for them.

Denise Marshall MBE is the Head of Services of Birth Companions—a unique charity working with women facing challenges and disadvantage in the perinatal period. The organisation began in 1996 after publicity about a woman from Holloway Prison being shackled in labour. Although the charity has grown and now works with women in the community in London, as well as working in four other prisons, the harsh environment of this early prison setting was a strong influence in shaping our ethos and way of working. Marshall's chapter explores how the unique Birth Companions way of working developed and what it means in practice. It will provide useful insights for others working with women with complex needs in the perinatal period, both in the statutory and voluntary sectors. More recently, Birth Companions have become aware of the literature around working in a trauma-informed way and have realised that this very much describes their approach with women, as well as how they look after their staff and volunteers.

Conclusion

Our book evolved through an acknowledgement of the multitude of complexities that some perinatal women and families face. We recognise that meeting the needs of women who may face disadvantage is essential to attaining excellence in the twenty-first century maternity care provision. There is an urgency for us to work together with women to address the shortcomings of maternity services as highlighted in MBRRACE 2020 [7]. Maternal mortality and stillbirth rates are increasing for women who are from Black, Asian and Minority ethnicities and for women experiencing extreme disadvantage. The need for us to work together in an unbiased way with women is crucial. Our book recognises the importance of third sector partnerships, working alongside women with lived experiences and bringing health professionals together. Health care professionals have a duty to be knowledgeable of those needs, acting with professionalism and compassion. Through our collective writing, we provide an exemplar for partnership working. Each chapter invites the reader to step into the shoes of the perinatal woman. We hope that through the knowledge gained and with compassion and advocacy, we can continue to provide the highest quality, non-judgemental care for women, whatever their social circumstances.

References

1. Knight M, Bunch K, Tuffnell D, Shakespeare J, Kotnis R, Kenyon S, Kurinczuk JJ, editors. on behalf of MBRRACE-UK. Saving lives, improving mothers' care—lessons learned to inform maternity care from the UK and Ireland Confidential Enquiries into Maternal Deaths and Morbidity 2016–18. Oxford: National Perinatal Epidemiology Unit, University of Oxford; 2020.
2. National Institute for Health and Care Excellence. Pregnancy and complex social factors: a model for service provision for pregnant women with complex social factors. NICE; Manchester; 2010.
3. National Institute for Health and Care Excellence. Pregnancy and complex social factors. Raising sensitive issues with pregnant women: training plan for maternity settings. NICE Clinical Guideline 110. 2011; https://www.nice.org.uk/guidance/cg110/resources/training-plan-pdf-544299230.
4. NHS England. National maternity review: better births improving outcomes of maternity services in England—a five year forward view for maternity care. London: NHS England. 2016.
5. Glover V, and O'Connor TG. Effects of antenatal stress and anxiety. Br J Psychiatry 180(5), 2002:389–91.
6. Knight M, Bunch K, Tuffnell D, Shakespeare J, Kotnis R, Kenyon S, Kurinczuk JJ, editors. on behalf of MBRRACE-UK. Saving lives, improving mothers' care—lessons learned to inform

maternity care from the UK and Ireland confidential enquiries into maternal deaths and morbidity 2016–18. Oxford: National Perinatal Epidemiology Unit, University of Oxford. 2020.
7. Knight M, Bunch K, Tuffnell D, Shakespeare J, Kotnis R, Kenyon S, Kurinczuk JJ, editors. on behalf of MBRRACE-UK. Saving Lives, Improving Mothers' Care - Lessons learned to inform maternity care from the UK and Ireland Confidential Enquiries into Maternal Deaths and Morbidity 2016-18. Oxford: National Perinatal Epidemiology Unit, University of Oxford 2020.

Overview of Complex Issues in Maternity Care in Relation to Current Guidance

Laura Abbott

Abstract

Women with complex social issues often experience a multitude of obstacles to maternity care. Often described by professionals as 'hard to reach' communities, it is contended that frequently, the responsibility lies with health-care experts not appropriately reaching such marginalised groups. Such barriers have been recognised in The National Institute for Health and Care Excellence (NICE) 'Pregnancy and Complex Social Factors: A Model for Service Provision for Pregnant Women with Complex Social Factors', first published in 2010. This chapter provides an overview of the current evidence, associated reports and guidance concerning the best practice and provision of care for pregnant women and new mothers' experiencing complex social issues (CSI). These include learning from the latest reports into maternal and neonatal death, guidance from evidence in relation to models of continuity of care for women, national guidance for best practice and recommendations from professional bodies and organisations. The chapter describes ways of managing sensitive issues and makes suggestions and recommendations for supporting communication skills with women experiencing CSI.

Keywords

Complex social issues · Barriers to care · Managing sensitive issues · Continuity of care · Pregnancy

L. Abbott (✉)
Department of Allied Health and Midwifery, University of Hertfordshire, Hatfield, Hertfordshire, UK
e-mail: l.abbott@herts.ac.uk

© Springer Nature Switzerland AG 2021   1
L. Abbott (ed.), *Complex Social Issues and the Perinatal Woman*,
https://doi.org/10.1007/978-3-030-58085-8_1

By the end of this chapter, the reader will:

- Understand the current key messages from reports and national guidance relating to the care of women experiencing complex social issues in maternity care.
- Have a greater understanding of the terminology in relation to complex social issues.
- Be able to consider ways in which to increase engagement and enhance communication with women enduring multiple and complex disadvantage.
- Reflect on ways of discussing sensitive issues with women who may be experiencing complex social circumstances and facing multiple disadvantages.

1.1   Introduction

Complex social factors may differ, in both type and frequency, across various local populations. Recommendations for improving maternity service delivery include the following areas [1]:

- Alcohol or drug misuse.
- Recent migrant or asylum seeker status.
- Difficulty reading or speaking English.
- Aged under 20.
- Domestic abuse.
- Poverty.
- Homelessness.

Women with social complexities often experience a multitude of barriers to maternity care. Often described as 'hard to reach' communities, it is argued that often health professionals are not trying sufficiently to reach marginalised groups [2]. Such barriers have been recognised in The National Institute for Health and Care Excellence (NICE) [1] 'Pregnancy and Complex Social Factors: A Model for Service Provision for Pregnant Women with Complex Social Factors', first published in 2010.

1.2   Pathways to Care

Midwifery 2020 Delivering Expectations [3] states that the complexities of women experiencing social diversity present clinical challenges in maternity care and have an increased risk for poor outcomes. Women with CSIs in maternity care may often present themselves booking their first antenatal appointment much later than most women or by presenting with a complex social history. Conversely, research has found that attending more antenatal appointments rather than what is currently recommended may lessen the occurrence of stillbirth [4]. NICE [1] recommends that midwives who lead the multidisciplinary team should work to improve health outcomes for women and babies experiencing multiple disadvantage. This might include facilitating education and staff training, alongside undertaking midwifery research to help provide vigorous evidence to ensure policy change as well as more practical pathways of local care.

The Nursing and Midwifery Council (NMC) expects all midwives to understand their role in recognising potential for harm, referring those who are at risk, working together with multi-agency teams and taking realistic steps to protect the woman from potential harm (NMC, 2019) [5]. The Saving Babies Lives Care Bundle [6] was developed by NHS England with the aim to reduce stillbirths and neonatal deaths. It encompasses two of the MBRRACE-UK recommendations, the Royal College of Obstetrics and Gynaecology (RCOG) 'Each Baby Counts [7]' and significant public health actions. It is recommended that interventions are targeted more specifically when women find services unapproachable or difficult to use [8]. The suggestion that any member of a multidisciplinary team should feel encouraged to contest decisions they feel may be inappropriate has been endorsed by professional organisations such as the RCOG, the Royal College of Midwives (RCM) and with reports such as 'Each Baby Counts' [7, 9]. The shedding of hierarchal structures and sense of feeling safe when speaking out should be adopted and transferable for any situation in maternity care where a woman may be at risk. Assuming accountability for the social welfare of the woman and family recognises that deviations from the midwives' scope of practice should be referred to specialist services (e.g., drug and alcohol services and/or social services).

1.3   Learning from Audits and Confidential Enquiries

The latest Mothers and Babies: Reducing Risk through Audits and Confidential Enquiries across the UK (MBRRACE-UK) [10] clearly demonstrates the consequences that having multiple complexities has and the need to ensure that susceptible groups receive tailored, timely care. Predictably, the development of mental health illness for women facing complex social issues is also well documented [11]. A case-control research study undertaken in 41 UK maternity units, measuring late stillbirth as its main outcome, has similarly demonstrated that pregnant women who experience CSIs such as domestic abuse, deprivation and extreme stress are at increased likelihood of having a stillborn baby [4].

There are substantial changes to maternity services in the UK proposed over the next 10 years, through the maternity transformation programme, via the National Health Service (NHS) Long Term Plan [12]. Meeting the needs of all women is essential in attaining excellence in the twenty-first-century care provision as outlined by NICE [1]. Articles three and eight of the Human Rights Act [13, 14] have a robust, legal foundation in the UK to protect against degrading treatment, defending the right to a private life and ensuring choice and dignity for all women. Birth Companions and Birthrites 'Holding it all together' research [15] offers useful explanations where the rights of women facing multiple disadvantages may be endangered. This includes professionals and services adopting a trauma-informed approach to care:

> *Respecting women's fundamental human rights to dignity, autonomy and equality should be central to the delivery of high quality, safe maternity care.* [15]

Health inequalities have been linked with maternity outcomes for families from Black, Asian and Minority Ethnic (BAME) backgrounds [16]. Maternal mortality and stillbirth rates are increasing for women who are from Black, Asian and Minority ethnicities and for women experiencing extreme disadvantage. The need to work together with women to address the shortcomings of maternity services is urgent, including the responses from Public Health England who have described racism as being especially noticeable during the COVID-19 pandemic [17]. The constellation of biases concept developed by MBRRACE [10] provides a useful visual info-graphic of the interlinking complexities pregnant or post-birth women face. The lay report states that 90% of the women who died endured multiple disadvantage, with 20% of women having had social services involvement [10].

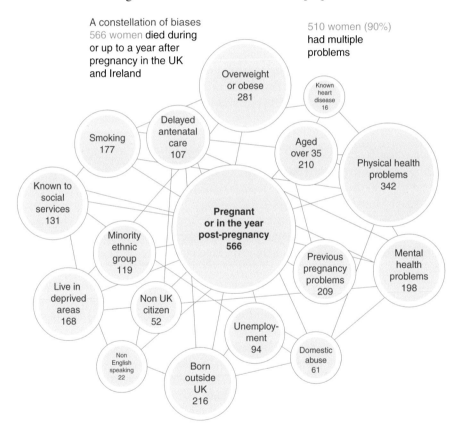

Systemic Biases due to pregnancy, health and other
issues prevent women with complex and multiple
problems receiving the care they need

Campaigns such as FIVEXMORE founded by two mothers to advocate and empower women to increase awareness of the statistics for BAME women and peti-tion the Government to improve maternity together with The Royal College of

Obstetricians and Gynaecologists are a powerful way of raising responsiveness to the MBRRACE statistics. Furthermore, inquiries such as those led by the charity and campaign group Birthrites [18–20] are calling to action inequalities and researching the reasons why Black women are five times more likely to die than their white counterparts [21].

Black and Asian women have a higher risk of dying in pregnancy

White women		7/100,000
Asian women	2x	13/100,000
Mixed ethnicity women	3x	23/100,000
Black women	5x	38/100,000

1.4 Hard to Reach or Professionals Not Reaching Hard Enough?

Non-engagement of maternity services is a well-known risk factor for adverse health outcomes in pregnancy [22]. Qualitative research challenges the concept of the 'late-booker' or non-attender in maternity services, giving reasons and examples for women not engaging as:

- Socio-economic reasons.
- Concealment (of pregnancy).
- Deficiency of knowledge about maternity health arrangements [23].

An audit into inner-city women experiencing socially complex lives [24] found that over 70% had not booked for maternity care by 12 weeks gestation and almost 89% primiparous women had less than the recommended number of antenatal appointments. An example of a CSI which has the potential to co-occur with other health or social challenges, such as substance misuse or mental health problems, is domestic abuse [25, 26]. It is recommended practice that midwives ensure routine enquiry for abuse, evaluating wellbeing and risk offering referral if required [27]. Models of care that are demonstrably successful, such as specialist continuity of care (CoC) teams, with midwifery expertise in CSIs, alongside improved communication skills, are important to ensure we reach women who may be vulnerable. Developing and enhancing communication skills, through training, reflection and clinical supervision, may be helpful to ensure team resilience. Templates such as the NICE Raising sensitive issues [28] are helpful with ensuring we maximise every contact with pregnant women [29].

Practical steps to improving the quality of care and services using NICE guidance [1] (Taken from https://intopractice.nice.org.uk/practical-stcps-improving-quality-of-care-services-using-nice-guidance/index.html).

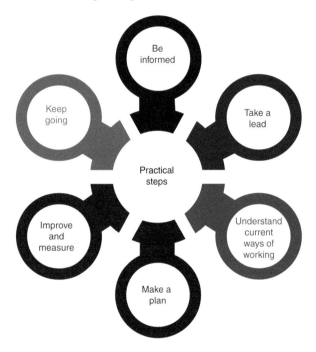

1.5   Improving Outcomes for Women and Babies through Continuity of Care

Continuity of care (CoC) is defined as midwifery care that is provided by the same midwife throughout the antenatal, labour and postnatal periods [30]. The Maternity Transformation Programme has been motivated by Better Births ambition for women to receive CoC, presently targeted for women who may need it most [30, 31]. An observational study compared outcomes for women with CSIs who received CoC to standard maternity care. Findings demonstrated a reduction in caesarean sections, antenatal and neonatal unit admissions and an increase in 'benefits and reduction of harm' for women [32]. The evidence for implementing CoC is also outlined in a Cochrane review where it was shown that women and babies received safer and improved outcomes, including a reduced likelihood in having a pre-term birth and improved maternal satisfaction throughout the pregnancy [33]. The evidence has led to NHS England ambitions to roll out CoC models across maternity services [34], with the NHS Long Term Plan [12] ambitious for 75% BAME women to experience CoC. The UK midwifery profession benefits from having a Chief Midwifery Officer, Professor Jacqueline Dunkley-Bent, who is committed to leading and facilitating the reduction of inequalities through ambitions of the rolling out of CoC for all women in the UK. Tackling health inequalities, Professor Dunkley-Bent describes and draws upon the concept of 'proportionate universalism' defined as an approach that:

> Balances targeted and universal public health perspectives through action proportionate to needs and levels of social vulnerability in a population. [35, 36]

The application of proportionate universalism to maternity services means implementing an intervention (such as CoC) where a good outcome can be facilitated for a woman and her baby [31].

The essence of midwifery philosophy focuses on pregnancy and birth as a physiological process, with empowerment, partnership and the locus of choice as central values [33, 37–39]. Indeed, promotion of choice and reduction of inequalities through using care models such as case loading and team midwifery have been recommended in England as part of the 2016 Better Births initiative, in the form of a 5-year plan to move toward continuity of midwifery care for all women [40]. Scoping reviews were prompted by the publication of the Marmot Review, Fair Society Healthy Lives, which considered health inequalities with special consideration for those who may be socially disadvantaged [41]. It is often understood that where there is one complex issue, there may be an overlapping of other multifaceted social issues, increasing the complexity of managing the care for the woman and necessitating multidisciplinary mixed-skill team working. The maternity transformation programme [42] calls for further individualised care.

Ten national programme work streams to supporting the implementation of Better Births [30].

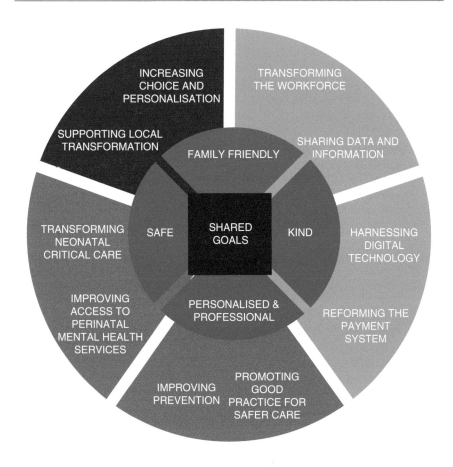

1.6   Understanding Women's Perspectives

A woman may have a spectrum of complexities, but she remains the expert of her own experiences and may have hidden challenges she may not wish to share. She may, for example, be practised in masking her mental health condition, may not wish to share her homeless status or the fact that she is on home detention curfew. Recommendations for policymakers and maternity care providers include the adoption of specialist services and challenging the prejudice and stigma that women facing extreme disadvantage may face [43].

Women who may be in a Minority (such as those with invisible disabilities, women in the criminal justice system) may not necessarily define themselves as having a complex need, yet there is a potential for being misunderstood, for being judged by being 'other' [44]. 'Othering' [45] is something that struck me during my own research – An autonomous identity is said to be essential in order to be 'related as one human being to another' [46]. Laing suggests that being depersonalised is 'dangerous', causing a potential existential crisis. We ask the reader to consider how we might inadvertently put women in boxes—examine our biases and seek to understand those who may be different to ourselves.

A Woman's Reflection

I sit in the waiting room, aware that the other women move away from me. I don't look like them. I don't smell like them, all freshly showered, nicely dressed and blooming with pregnancy. All my life my body has been used and bears the bruises and scars from others. The drugs numb and take the pain away, momentarily. The cigarettes keep my hands occupied so I don't pick at the scars. The alcohol is cheap but helps me forget a childhood of trauma. I hear the midwife call my name as I disappear back outside, but I cannot face her today. She writes DNA across my maternity notes.

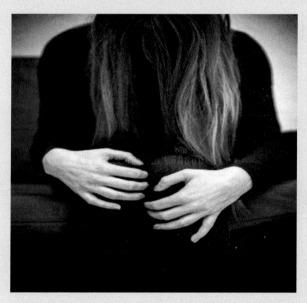

Trust in the person providing care is essential if the woman is going to feel able to share and disclose the challenges she is facing [15, 47]. The importance of the midwife/woman relationship and compassion, sensitivity and warmth are essential components for such a trusting relationship [48]. The evidence that having continuity of care from a specialist known midwife not only enhances the woman's overall experience but empowers women [43].

Communicating Sensitive Issues Adapted from NICE Ten Tips for Raising Sensitive Issues Guidance [8, 28]:
- **Privacy**
  - Prepare the setting and ensure no interruptions.
- **Perception**
  - Listen to the words she chooses (e.g., using negative, disempowered language "he goes out, I don't go out"), and witness how she interacts with her partner/family if present (e.g., does she seem nervous, and is she at ease? [28])
- **Space**
  - Allow time for responses. Be comfortable with silences. Ask open questions.
- **Sensitivity**
  - Respect her responses, and understand that she may not wish to share information. Build trust.
- **Compassion**
  - Show empathy, and validate her concerns. Avoid assumptions, minimising or comparisons.
- **Judgements**
  - Avoid making judgements about lifestyle choices or assumptions about her circumstances.
- **Confidentiality**
  - Honesty from the outset about confidentiality limitations (e.g., child protection). Adopt a methodical approach to how you phrase this.
- **Reflection**
  - Learn to summarise what the woman has said to verify understanding.
- **Planning**
  - Always in partnership with the woman and coordinated with the multidisciplinary team.

National Institute for Health and Care Excellence. (2011). Pregnancy and Complex Social Factors. Raising Sensitive Issues with Pregnant Women: Training Plan for Maternity Settings. NICE Clinical Guideline 110. Retrieved November 18th, 2020 from https://www.nice.org.uk/guidance/cg110/resources/training-plan-pdf-544,299,230

1.7   Conclusion

This chapter has outlined key messages relating to the care of women experiencing CSIs and has encouraged reflection on potential judgements. It has endorsed the policy recommendations from continuity of care pathways that target specific groups such as women from Black, Asian and ethnic minority women communities and those experiencing disadvantage. It has drawn upon evidence from research and latest reports into maternal mortality and suggested ways of communicating sensitively. There is an urgency for us to work together with women to address the shortcomings of maternity services as highlighted in MBRRACE 2020 [10]. Maternal mortality and stillbirth rates are increasing for women who are from Black, Asian and Minority ethnicities and for women experiencing extreme disadvantage. The need for us to work together in an unbiased way with women is crucial. Our book recognises the importance of third sector partnerships, working alongside women with lived experiences and bringing health professionals together. Health-care professionals have a duty to be knowledgeable of those needs, acting with professionalism and compassion.

References

1. National Institute for Health and Care Excellence. Pregnancy and complex social factors: a model for service provision for pregnant women with complex social factors. Manchester; 2010. https://www.nice.org.uk/guidance/cg110
2. Mason T, Carlisle C, Watkins C. Stigma and social exclusion in healthcare. Psychology Press; 2001.
3. Department of Health, Social Services and Public Safety & Department of Health, Social Services and Public Safety. Midwifery 2020: delivering expectations. London: Midwifery 2020 Programme, DoH & DHSSPS; 2010.
4. Heazell AE, Budd J, Smith LK, Li M, Cronin R, Bradford B, McCowan LM, Mitchell EA, Stacey T, Roberts D and Thompson JM. Associations between social and behavioural factors and the risk of late stillbirth–findings from the Midland and North of England Stillbirth case-control study. BJOG: Int J Obstet Gynaecol 2020.
5. Nursing and Midwifery Council. Midwives rules and standards 2019. London: NMC; 2019.
6. Morton VH and Morris RK. Overview of the saving babies lives care bundle version 2. Obstet Gynaecol Reprod Med. 2020.
7. NHS England. Saving babies lives: a care bundle for reducing stillbirth. London: NHS England; 2016. p. 30.
8. NICE. Pregnancy and complex social factors overview. NICE. Retrieved on 19th January 2021 from http://pathways.nice.org.uk/pathways/pregnancy-and-complexsocialfactors; 2014.
9. https://www.rcog.org.uk/en/guidelines-research-services/audit-quality-improvement/each-baby-counts/reports-updates/2019-progress-report/learning-points/
10. Knight M, Bunch K, Tuffnell D, Shakespeare J, Kotnis R, Kenyon S, Kurinczuk JJ, on behalf of MBRRACE-UK. Saving lives, improving mothers' care—lessons learned to inform maternity care from the UK and Ireland confidential enquiries into maternal deaths and morbidity 2016–18. Oxford: National Perinatal Epidemiology Unit, University of Oxford; 2020.
11. Department of Health. Annual report of the chief medical officer 2014. The Health of the 51%: Women. https://www.gov.uk/government/uploads/system/uploads/attachment_data/file/595439/CMO_annual_report_2014.pdf; 2014.
12. The NHS Long-Term Plan. https://www.longtermplan.nhs.uk/wp-content/uploads/2019/08/nhs-long-term-plan-version-1.2.pdf [Accessed 20th December 2020].
13. Schiller R. Why human rights in childbirth matter. Pinter and Martin; 2016.
14. Citizens Advice Bureau. https://www.citizensadvice.org.uk/law-and-courts/civil-rights/human-rights/what-rights-are-protected-under-the-human-rights-act/your-right-not-to-be-tortured-or-treated-in-an-inhuman-way/; [accessed 26.09.2020]; 2019.
15. Birthrights and Birth Companions (2019). Holding it all together: understanding how far the human rights of woman facing disadvantage are respected during pregnancy, birth and postnatal care. London [online].

16. Khan Z. Ethnic health inequalities in the UK's maternity services: a systematic literature review. Br J Midwifery., February 2021. 2020;29:2.
17. Public Health England. Beyond the data, understanding the impact of Covid-19 on BAME groups. 2020. https://assets.publishing.service.gov.uk/government/uploads/system/uploads/attachment_data/file/892376/COVID_stakeholder_engagement_synthesis_beyond_the_data.pdf (accessed 10 February 2021).
18. https://www.fivexmore.com/
19. https://www.birthrights.org.uk/2021/02/07/new-inquiry-to-drive-action-on-racial-injustice-in-maternity-care/
20. https://www.rcog.org.uk/en/news/campaigns-and-opinions/race-equality-taskforce/five-steps-for-healthcare-professionals/
21. https://www.npeu.ox.ac.uk/assets/downloads/mbrrace-uk/reports/maternal-report-2020/MBRRACE-UK_Maternal_Report_2020_-_Lay_Summary_v10.pdf
22. Raatikainen K, Heiskanen N, Heinonen S. Under-attending free antenatal care is associated with adverse pregnancy outcomes. BMC Public Health. 2007;7(1):1–8.
23. Haddrill R, Jones GL, Mitchell CA, Anumba DO. Understanding delayed access to antenatal care: a qualitative interview study. BMC Pregnancy Childbirth. 2014;14(1):1–4.
24. Rayment-Jones H, Butler E, Miller C, Nay C, O'Dowd J. A multisite audit to assess how women with complex social factors access and engage with maternity services. Midwifery. 2017;52:71–7.
25. National Institute for Health and Care Excellence. (2014). Domestic Violence and Abuse: Multi-Agency Working. Public Health Guideline. Published: 26 February 2014. Retrieved November 25th 2020 https://www.nice.org.uk/guidance/ph50/resources/domestic-violence-and-abuse-multiagency-working-1996411687621
26. World Health Organisation. Responding to intimate partner violence and sexual violence against women. Taking Action and Generating Evidence. 2013. http://apps.who.int/iris/bitstream/10665/44350/1/9789241564007_eng.pdf?ua=1
27. Department of Health. Responding to domestic violence. a resource for health pofessionals. 2017 Retrieved November, 23, 2017 from https://www.gov.uk/government/uploads/system/uploads/attachment_data/file/597435/DometicAbuseGuidance.pdf
28. National Institute for Health and Care Excellence. Pregnancy and complex social factors. Raising sensitive issues with pregnant women: training plan for maternity settings. NICE Clinical Guideline 110. 2011 Retrieved November 18th 2020 from https://www.nice.org.uk/guidance/cg110/resources/training-plan-pdf-544299230
29. National Health Service. London maternal deaths 2016 Review October 2017. NHS London Clinical Networks. 2017. Retrieved November, 29, 2017 from http://www.londonscn.nhs.uk/wp-content/uploads/2016/08/London-maternal-mortality-report-2015.pdf
30. Cumberledge J. National maternity review. Better births. London: NHS; 2016.
31. NHS England. Maternity transformation programme. www.england.nhs.uk/mat-transformation. 2017.
32. Rayment-Jones HT, Murrells T, Sandall J. An investigation of the relationship between the caseload model of midwifery for socially disadvantaged women and childbirth outcomes using routine data—a retrospective, observational study. Midwifery. 2015;31(4):409–17.
33. Sandall J, Soltani H, Gates S, Shennan A, Devane D. Midwife-led continuity models versus other models of care for childbearing women. Cochrane Database Syst Rev. 2016;4
34. NHS England. Implementing better births: continuity of carer. 2017. https://www.england.nhs.uk/publication/implementingbetter-births-continuity-of-carer
35. Shipstone RA, Young J, Kearney L, Thompson J. Applying a social exclusion framework to explore the relationship between sudden unexpected deaths in infancy (SUDI) and social vulnerability. Front Public Health. 2020;8:629.
36. Harron K, Gilbert R, Fagg J, Guttmann A, van der Meulen J. Associations between pre-pregnancy psychosocial risk factors and infant outcomes: a population-based cohort study in England. Lancet Public Health. 2021;6(2):e97–105.

37. Sandall J. Choice, continuity and control: changing midwifery, towards a sociological perspective. Midwifery. 1995;11(4):201–9.
38. McCourt C, Stevens T, Sandall J, Brodie P. Working with women: developing continuity of care in practice. The New Midwifery: Science and Sensitivity in Practice; 2006. p. 141–65.
39. Mander R. The partnership model. Chapter 14. In: Bryar R, Sinclair M, editors. Theory for midwifery practice. 2nd ed. Basingstoke: Palgrave Macmillan; 2011. p. 304–17.
40. Cumberledge J. National maternity review. Better births: improving outcomes for maternity services in England: a five year forward view for maternity care. London: NHS; 2016. https://www.england.nhs.uk/wp-content/uploads/2017/12/implementing-better-births.pdf [accessed 22.12.2021]
41. Marmot MG. Fair society, healthy lives: the marmot review. Executive summary: strategic review of health inequalities in England Post-2010. 2010.
42. Department of Health. Safer maternity care the national maternity safety strategy-progress and next steps. 2017. https://assets.publishing.service.gov.uk/government/uploads/system/uploads/attachment_data/file/662969/Safer_maternity_care_-_progress_and_next_steps.pdf (accessed 04 February 2021).
43. McLeish J, Redshaw M. Maternity experiences of mothers with multiple disadvantages in England: a qualitative study. Women Birth. 2019;32(2):178–84.
44. Johnson JL, Bottorff JL, Browne AJ, Grewal S, Hilton BA, Clarke H. Othering and being Othered in the context of health care services. Health Commun. 2004;16(2):255–71.
45. Canales MK. Othering: toward an understanding of difference. Adv Nurs Sci. 2000;22(4):16–31.
46. Laing R. The divided self: an existential study in sanity and madness (Vol. 731) Penguin UK; 1960.
47. Francis R Report of the mid staffordshire nhs foundation trust public inquiry, Executive Summary; 2013.
48. Byrom S, Ménage D. 7 Sustained by compassion. Sustainability, Midwifery and Birth. 2020.

Trauma-Informed Care of Perinatal Women

2

Naomi Delap

Abstract

The potential for women to be re-traumatised is heightened during pregnancy and childbirth, especially for women who may have been survivors of sexual abuse. Trauma-informed maternity services should be targeted, holistic, universal and designed collaboratively and holistically with stakeholders including women with lived experience. Trauma-informed care is a way of understanding and supporting people whose lives have been shaped adversely by traumatic events. This chapter defines trauma, which are often linked to Adverse Childhood Experiences (A.C.Es). The implementation of trauma-informed care in the perinatal period in maternity and mental health services includes issues around: choice and consent, improving care, integrated care and the care of staff. Women's experiences are central to the discussions about the impact upon the pregnant woman and the new mother, utilising the latest evidence. The reader is encouraged to consider birth-related trauma and understand women's perspectives through summaries of their experiences. It should be assumed that many women will engage with maternity services without disclosing their experiences of sexual abuse. The foundations of good practice in adopting a trauma-informed approach to care draw upon women's lived experience. Charities and Non-Governmental Organisations (NGOs) have an important part to play in supporting women alongside maternity service providers. The reader is encouraged to consider the fact that women may not wish to share their experiences, yet still need their potential distress addressed. This chapter inspires the reader to reflect upon the five values suggested for ensuring TIC approaches (Safety, Trustworthiness, Choice, Collaboration and Empowerment).

N. Delap (✉)
Birth Companions, London, UK

© Springer Nature Switzerland AG 2021
L. Abbott (ed.), *Complex Social Issues and the Perinatal Woman*,
https://doi.org/10.1007/978-3-030-58085-8_2

Keywords

Trauma-informed approaches · Trauma-informed care · Adverse childhood experiences · Birth trauma · Trauma-informed maternity services

"It comes down to the question of not 'what's wrong with you? [but]... what happened to you...?'"
   Oprah Winfrey, Treating Childhood Trauma, CBS News [1]
   "Last year I met a woman who told me that, apart from the day she was raped, giving birth to her child was the most traumatic day of her life. Throughout labour and her baby son's first few hours of life, images of her rapist's face and of the rape itself continuously flashed through her mind. With vaginal examinations being carried out, contractions forcing her out of control of her own body, and strangers constantly touching her without her consent, she began remembering and reliving the rape that she thought she had left behind many years before...
   Throughout her pregnancy...[she]...had avoided antenatal appointments. She was frightened of being so physically out of control and of experiencing flashbacks of what had happened. She didn't know how to tell staff what was running through her mind so she simply avoided all pregnancy check-ups... For those first, crucial, hours of her child's life she couldn't bond with him because she was too busy trying to keep herself sane."
   Pavan Amara, founder of the My Body Back Project [2]

Trauma-informed care (TIC) is a way of understanding and supporting people whose lives have been shaped adversely by traumatic events. While the concept of trauma-informed care has gained significant traction in certain services in the UK such as drug and alcohol and mental health and has influenced pockets of practice with perinatal women, it has yet to inform maternity services and the care of perinatal women in a systematic, systemic way. Yet the evidence suggests that a trauma-informed approach might be of *particular* relevance to maternity services and that positive outcomes for mothers, babies, families and maternal health professionals could be significant if this avenue of care was investigated.

This chapter will discuss the adverse effect of childhood and adult experiences of trauma and how gendered experiences of trauma can amplify and compound its impact. It will explore the effects of trauma on women during pregnancy, birth and the postpartum period, examine existing trauma-related practice in maternal health and look at the case for the introduction of a trauma-informed approach within maternity services.

2.1   What Is Trauma?

Definitions of trauma vary, but a useful summary describes trauma as "an event, series of events, or set of circumstances that is experienced by an individual as physically or emotionally harmful or life threatening and that has lasting adverse effects on the individual's functioning and mental, physical, social, emotional, or spiritual well-being" [3]. Although childhood experiences of trauma are particularly significant in shaping the course of individuals' lives, many adults will also experience traumatic events that go on to affect their later experiences adversely. Some are more likely to have these experiences in adulthood as a result of the factors that shaped their childhoods; others will experience trauma for the first time in adulthood.

Traumatic experiences are a normal part of most individual's lives, and many people respond to them with resilience. However, there are some types of traumatic events and some ways of experiencing them that can lead to a person's increased likelihood of suffering from ill health, being affected adversely by social factors and choosing harmful behaviours throughout their life, and can even impact negatively on their children. In particular, a growing body of evidence has established a correlation between multiple traumatic experiences in childhood and health-harming behaviour in later life and that women suffer disproportionately from some severe types of trauma which correlate strongly with multiple disadvantage.

2.1.1   Adverse Childhood Experiences

The term adverse childhood experiences (ACEs) refers to traumatic or stressful events experienced during the course of childhood. While precise definitions of ACEs vary, most sources agree that the ACEs that harm a child directly include physical, verbal or sexual abuse and physical or emotional neglect. ACEs that affect the environment in which a child grows up include parents separating, domestic violence, mental illness, drug and alcohol use and parental imprisonment [4, 5]. Physiological and biomolecular studies show how childhood exposure to chronic stress can influence changes to the development of the immune, nervous and endocrine systems [6]. These changes result in impaired cognitive, social and emotional functions and increased allostatic load (the "cost" of the body's adaptation to repeated or chronic stress that can accelerate disease processes) [7]. The stress children incur as a result of ACEs can impact negatively on the development of their ability to learn, think rationally and regulate their behaviours. The more ACEs a child experiences, the greater the chance the child will experience health and/or social problems in later life [4, 5].

Multiple ACEs and Incidence of Health-Harming Behaviours
The English ACE population study (2014) found that:

- 53% of the population in England had experienced 0 ACEs.
- 23% had experienced 1 ACE.
- 15% had experienced 2–3 ACEs.
- 9% had experienced 4+ ACEs.

The study discovered a strong correlation between those who had experienced multiple ACEs and the increased risk of developing health harming behaviours. Compared with people with no ACEs, those with 4+ ACEs are:

- 2 times more likely to currently binge drink and have a poor diet
- 3 times more likely to smoke
- 5 times more likely to have had sex when under 16 years old
- 6 times more likely to have had or caused a teenage pregnancy
- 7 times more likely to have been involved in violence in the last year
- 11 times more likely to have used heroin/crack/been imprisoned [8]

It is instructive to view the data above through the lens of maternity services, leading as it does to insight into and understanding of the factors that may contribute to teenage pregnancy rates and health-harming behaviours during the perinatal period. It has also been used in understanding the background of trauma in the lives of a large number of women who experience the repeated removal of their children into care (see below).

2.1.2 Women's Experiences of Trauma

Women suffer disproportionately from certain types of trauma, and the impact of this trauma is significant. In 2016, the Office for National Statistics included for the first time questions about respondents' experiences of childhood abuse. It showed that 6% of women in England and Wales experienced four types of abuse in childhood: psychological abuse, physical abuse, sexual assault and witnessing domestic violence or abuse; compared to 2% of men. 14% of women experienced three types of abuse in childhood [9].

Hidden Hurt: Violence, abuse and disadvantage in the lives of women, a recent study [10] utilising data from the Adult Psychiatric Morbidity Study 2014 [11], demonstrated that about 5% women in England have experienced extensive physical and sexual violence and abuse across their life course starting in childhood, compared to 1% of men. These 1.2 million women have been sexually abused as children or severely beaten by a parent or carer, and many have been raped as adults and suffered severe abuse from a partner including being choked, strangled or threatened with a weapon. A further 3% of women have experienced extensive physical violence from a partner in adulthood.

The study shows that women with extensive experience of physical and sexual violence will be far more likely to experience disadvantage and inequality in other areas of their lives, including physical and mental ill health and disability, substance dependence, poverty and debt, poor living conditions and homelessness and discrimination. In the group that had experienced extensive physical/sexual violence, over half (54%) met the diagnostic criteria for at least one common mental disorder

(CMD), 16% screened positive for post-traumatic stress disorder (PTSD) and 15% had three or more mental disorders. To make matters worse, the evidence showed that most women were not receiving treatment or support for their mental health issues. At the time of the survey, the majority of women experiencing these very high levels of mental ill-health (75%) were receiving neither medication nor counselling for a mental health problem.

It is clear how women's experiences of extreme trauma, particularly those that start during childhood, take a toll on their lives. We can extrapolate from the data above that the vast majority of women who have experienced extensive physical and sexual violence as children and who go on to have children will pass through maternity services. A significant number of women giving birth will therefore do so with a background of trauma and its attendant impact. Those from low-income and high "psychosocial risk" groups are *most* likely to have experienced lifetime trauma [12]. Another lens through which to view this group of women is that of multiple disadvantage: women who report three or more complex social factors during pregnancy are at a higher risk of having experienced trauma before pregnancy, and of experiencing trauma during pregnancy [13].

Pregnancy and childbirth is a period which survivors of the trauma of childhood and adult sexual abuse may find particularly challenging, in which the potential for women to be re-traumatised is significant. Yet research has identified that many women are reluctant to disclose their experiences (although they wanted their distress to be noticed and addressed) and that maternity care professionals were often reluctant to elicit disclosure because it required a response from them that they did not have the skills, knowledge or time to give [14]. Thus, it should be assumed that many women will engage with maternity services without disclosing their experiences of sexual abuse.

2.2 The Impact of Trauma during the Perinatal Period

The impact of trauma experienced by women during pregnancy on their outcomes and those of their babies is well documented. Women whose lives have been shaped by trauma are at an even higher risk: they are more likely both to experience trauma during pregnancy and to have their lifetime trauma impact negatively during the perinatal period. As we will see, experiences of trauma have established as a risk factor for a range of vulnerabilities and poor outcomes during the perinatal period including adverse reproductive and obstetric outcomes, perinatal depression, PTSD and problematic attachment, and some research points to the intergenerational transmission of trauma.

2.2.1 Increased Risks of Adverse Outcomes

Toxic stress (severe, prolonged or repetitive stress) during pregnancy is found to "increase significantly the levels of the hormone cortisol in the mother's body which, when it crosses the placenta, can affect the health of the baby, brain development, emotional attachment and early parenting interactions" [15]. As we saw from the evidence on ACEs and women's experiences of lifetime trauma, it is likely that previous experiences of trauma will correlate with an increased risk women will experience trauma during pregnancy. Recent research suggests that lifetime trauma history, and childhood experience of trauma in particular, is associated with potentially adverse reproductive outcomes that range from increased risk of being at a younger age at first pregnancy [16], a higher number of pregnancies [17], a history of miscarriage [18] to a magnification of the prediction of low birthweight [19]. Lifetime trauma experiences increased significantly the risk of both lifetime and antenatal depression and anxiety. These in turn are linked with a range of adverse psychiatric and physiological outcomes for mothers and children [17].

2.2.2 Birth-Related Trauma

It is estimated that 3% of women who give birth go on to develop postnatal post-traumatic stress disorder (PTSD) [20], around 20,000 new cases each year in the UK [21]. Symptoms of PTSD include re-experiencing the trauma through flash-backs and nightmares; avoidance of trauma-related situations, negative cognitions and mood; and arousal. The impact of PTSD can be significant: women might find it hard to bond with their babies; they may avoid contact with medical professionals or other new mothers because they act as a reminder of the birth, leading to missed appointments or social isolation; anxiety and irritability can lead to relationship problems; women might be reluctant to have another baby, and subsequent pregnancies can trigger the trauma of the initial birth [21].

While women of all types and backgrounds can experience postnatal PTSD as a result of events in childbirth, there is growing evidence that women who have experienced trauma in their lives *before* pregnancy (with the associated impacts outlined above) are at a greater risk of developing PTSD and find it harder to resolve. A recent meta-analytic review of the aetiology of PTSD after birth proposes a model that demonstrates how risk factors in pregnancy, such as a history of trauma and sexual abuse and previous psychological problems, interact with birth events to determine experiences of birth as traumatic and shape women's subsequent responses. Risk factors associated with birth include a high level of intervention and complication, perceived threat, dissociation, high levels of negative emotion and lack of support. Postpartum risk factors that contribute to maintaining symptoms of PTSD were detailed as poor support, additional stress and maladaptive coping. Understanding how existing vulnerabilities contribute to the risk of developing birth-related PTSD can inform the development of screening, prevention and targeted support during and after birth and should inform psychological assessment and treatment of postpartum PTSD.

Birth trauma also takes its toll on maternity staff. According to a 2016 survey of midwives, almost all had experienced a TPE or traumatic perinatal event (421 out of 464 respondents) with an average of seven events per midwife; at least one in 20 had experienced symptoms of PTSD; 35% had seriously considered leaving the profession after a TPE and 12% had taken time off work [22]. Research in this area suggests that midwives are not receiving the support they need in order to address the impact of birth trauma: in a qualitative investigation of the experience and impact of traumatic perinatal event experiences in midwives [23], those interviewed perceived support from supervisors and senior colleagues to be absent or inadequate. There is little research investigating the interaction between a background of personal experience of trauma and experience of birth-related trauma in maternity staff.

Mothers Who Experience Separation from their Babies
Many maternal healthcare professionals will experience the difficult role of caring for a perinatal woman whose contact with social services results in her separation from her baby. Understanding the background of trauma that women in these situations have frequently lived through, the traumatic nature of separation itself and what women say about their experiences of maternity services during this time will be essential to providing trauma-informed care.

Vulnerable Mothers and Recurrent Care Proceedings
Vulnerable Mothers and Recurrent Care Proceedings (2017) [24] was a groundbreaking research project: the first comprehensive study focussing on birth mothers who experienced recurrent care proceedings in England. Based on a range of data from national electronic records held by the Children and Family Court Advisory and Support Service (CAFCASS), to court files and in-depth qualitative interviews with birth mothers, the study set out to explore the backgrounds and experiences of women who experienced the removal of at least one child and were involved in at least one further care proceeding; and many of whom had lost multiple children to public care and adoption. Despite the very distressing impact of these proceedings on families and extremely high cost to public services, the scale of this problem was unknown until the publication of this research, and there had been no systematic analysis of the reasons behind women's return to court.

Using court case files, the study explored the adverse childhood experiences (ACEs) of 354 birth mothers. This work demonstrated that mothers in this group had experienced much higher levels of childhood adversity and exposure to trauma than the general population. Amongst the findings:

- 56% of mothers had experienced four or more ACEs.
- There was a very high prevalence of abuse and neglect in their childhoods: 66% had experienced neglect, 67% had experienced emotional abuse, 52% had experienced physical abuse and 53% had experienced sexual abuse.
- Around 40% of mothers had been looked after children, and around 14% had spent time not living with their parents through an informal care arrangement.

This research is of particular relevance to those caring for perinatal women. In the population-level data, it was found that 10.8% of children were aged under 4 weeks when court proceedings were issued, increasing to 47.3% and 53.3% at the first and second repeat proceedings, respectively.

How did the women involved in this study experience this very significant trauma of losing their children to public care and adoption, and how were they supported through this? Through qualitative interviews, the study found:

- Following the removal of their children, women experienced acute and enduring grief.
- Resolving this grief was complicated by women's feelings of anger towards children's services and of not being sufficiently understood or helped.
- Many women talked about symptoms of mental ill-health that should have been responded to professionally.
- Due to this grief, and lack of support, women often found themselves in a situation that was far worse than before their child was removed.
- Mothers' own experiences of the care system meant their children's futures in public care or with adopters caused them great anxiety.

This evidence demonstrates the background of trauma informing the experiences of a great number of women who lose their children to the care system; the high number that do so very close to the birth of a child; and the high levels of unresolved trauma women experienced as a result of losing their child to the care system.

Improving Women's Experiences of Maternity Services

The experiences of perinatal women whose babies were removed or who were at risk of having their babies removed during the perinatal period were explored further in *Making Better Births a reality for women with multiple disadvantages, a qualitative peer research study exploring perinatal women's experiences of care and services in north-east London* [13] (2018). The research identified significant gaps in services and gave some useful indications on the practical ways in which those involved with women's care could improve their experiences, particularly after the removal of the baby:

"One woman, whose baby was taken into care, described how she felt she might have been offered more support during pregnancy:

"...I would like to have had proper support really, but thinking of it, I never really got that support to be honest with you...".

"Another woman knew from very early on in pregnancy that her baby would be taken into care but did not receive support around this from maternity services during pregnancy or at birth.

"To me it was all just about taking the baby you know, really. They never really asked, really, you know, me being sad...".

"...in another case, a midwife not only remained a constant presence in the mother's pregnancy but also supported her through child protection meetings and an eventual court hearing. There it was agreed that her unborn child would be removed due to domestic violence concerns...This midwife was present until the birth of the baby, but was not involved when the baby was taken into care at 4 days old and no further midwifery support was available. The mother did have a routine physical check up with the GP but was offered no psychological support to help her manage her emotions following the removal of her baby...".

"Women at risk of having their baby removed into care expressed a desire for honest information and practical help. Many needed preparation for what was to come and said they would like bereavement counselling to be offered in pregnancy. One woman asked for "a grief counsellor"..." [13].

The report's recommendations included developing a specialist midwifery role to support women at risk of or going through separation [13].

2.3   Trauma-Informed Care

I've learned that people will forget what you said, people will forget what you did, but people will never forget how you made them feel. (Maya Angelou)

The information above demonstrates the high prevalence of trauma in the histories of a significant proportion of childbearing women and shows how these histories can impact negatively on women's experiences of care during the perinatal period and on the outcomes of mothers and children. How does the type of care a woman receives during the perinatal period impact on her experiences in relation to trauma, and the outcomes of her and her baby; and what would an effective model of care for these perinatal women look like? This section will look at current trauma-informed practice with perinatal women and what these limited examples tell us about the potential impact of such an approach. It will propose that maternity services *as whole systems* would benefit from adapting their ways of working to equip them to provide trauma-informed care. It will explore the argument that a trauma-informed maternity system not only would be better at caring for perinatal women affected by trauma but would contribute to the support and retention of staff and that the positive impact of a trauma-informed approach would have far-reaching effects on *all* women and families in the care of maternity services.

2.3.1   Current Trauma-Informed Practice with Perinatal Women

There are currently pockets of trauma-informed and trauma-specific practice in the UK for perinatal women who have experienced trauma.

Birth Companions

Birth Companions is a charity that works to improve the lives of women and babies who experience severe disadvantage during the perinatal period. The charity uses a trauma-informed framework for the practical services it offers women, which include antenatal courses, birth support and a mother and baby group.

Research done by Birth Companions to map the past experiences and present needs of perinatal women experiencing severe disadvantage confirms the high incidence of trauma experienced by women with multiple needs (three or more co-occurring complex social factors) [25]. Birth Companions does not use routine enquiry into women's previous experiences of trauma, but there is such a strong correlation between severe disadvantage and past trauma that a trauma-informed model is essential.

Read Chap. 13 for a detailed information about Birth Companions' trauma-informed model of care.

My Body Back Maternity Clinic

Started in 2014, the My Body Back Project supports people who have experienced rape or sexual violence to start to love and care for their bodies again. The My Body Back Maternity Clinic at Barts NHS Healthcare Trust in north-east London is the world's first designated maternity clinic for rape survivors.

Contributing to the design of the clinic, women who had experienced sexual assault described how memories and flashbacks of being raped were triggered during pregnancy and labour. Sometimes, women's bonding with their babies was affected, and other women decided they couldn't breastfeed for fear of being triggered. Women felt very isolated and unable to tell anyone how they were feeling, and so maternity staff didn't understand why they were, for example, so upset during vaginal examinations or particularly emotional or dissociated during labour. Staff were not always sympathetic or caring in these situations; some women were told to "grow up" by staff who thought they were being excessively emotional. Understandably, women were often reluctant to engage with services after the birth of their babies. There weren't felt enough specialist maternity services for women who had experienced sexual violence.

My Body Back's maternity clinic offers a specialist pathway for women and birthing people who have experienced sexual violence which includes pre-conception support, pregnancy care and examinations, antenatal classes, breastfeeding advice, specialist advice on mental wellbeing during labour, post-natal examinations and post-natal mental health support.

http://www.mybodybackproject.com

The UK Survivor Mums' Companion

Designed to support pregnant women with a history of childhood trauma, the UK Survivor Mums' Companions is a telephone-based programme that provides women in the Blackpool area with information, emotional support and the opportunity to learn new skills. Aimed at survivors of physical, sexual and emotional abuse or neglect, the service addresses the needs of women who are at risk of or experiencing PTSD symptoms during pregnancy and addresses women's fears around parenting and bonding.

The UK Survivor Mums' Companion was adapted from a US programme designed by Julia Seng and Mickey Sperlich, academics who have pioneered research into and practical approaches to the provision of trauma-informed care in the perinatal period [26].

https://blackpoolbetterstart.org.uk/pregnant-under1/survivor-mums-companion/

2.3.2   The Positive Impact of Trauma-Informed Care

Evaluation of the impact of small pockets of current trauma-informed practice and research looking at experiences of maternity care of groups with high levels of lifetime trauma gives an insight into the potential value of a system-wide trauma-informed approach. External evaluations of Birth Companions' Community Link service (which offers women facing multiple disadvantage individual support through pregnancy, birth and the postnatal period) highlight the organisation's unique trauma-informed approach, "Birth Companions' emphasis on building relationships through an informal and caring approach allowed them to gain trust where other services were unable to do so [27]", and the positive impact on women's experiences and outcomes which ranged from protecting against perinatal anxiety and depression [28] to the potential to improve women's birth outcomes [29].

Research into the maternity care experienced by survivors of childhood sexual abuse showed that "demonstrating respect and enabling women to retain control is crucial in providing sensitive care...Trusting relationships nurtured by open communication are crucial in helping women to feel safe. Getting to know women may alert midwives to cues that suggest that all is not well, even if the cause remains hidden..." [14].

A number of studies have pointed to the benefits of midwifery-led continuity of carer models, which hold the potential to address fear and distrust of services [25] and promote trusting relationships [14]. A compassionate and non-judgemental approach made a significant difference to women: "kindness (or lack of it) could shape people's experiences profoundly..."and where continuity of carer models were not available "...lack of continuity of care could be mitigated by a consistently caring approach" [25].

2.3.3 What Would Trauma-Informed Maternity Services Look like?

A trauma-informed approach is increasingly informing areas of service provision such as substance misuse and mental health, in which service users are more likely than the general population to have experienced trauma, and indeed whose challenges may have resulted in part or largely from their past experiences of trauma. This approach has yet to be transposed as a whole systems model to a universal service such as maternity, but there are many reasons to explore the potential of such a model. While the kind of trauma-informed specialist services outlined above do highly regarded work with small numbers of women, they cannot possibly address the needs of the large numbers of women across the country who have experienced significant trauma. Even while supported by specialist services, many women are re-traumatised during and through their contact with maternity services. Many women will pass through maternity services without ever disclosing their experiences of trauma, limiting their access to specialist services while leaving them at risk from re-traumatisation. The perinatal period represents both a challenge and a great opportunity for women with lifetime experiences of trauma and the maternity services working with them. Trauma-informed maternity services could be a framework through which to address the challenges and maximise the opportunities to improve outcomes for these women and their babies.

Foundations of Trauma-Informed Practice
There are many different definitions of the basic tenets and principles of trauma-informed care. One organisation that has been at the forefront of developing and promoting trauma-informed models of care in the USA is the Substance Abuse and Mental Health Services Administration (SAMHSA), a branch of the US Department of Health and Human Services. SAMHSA proposed that a trauma-informed approach "should incorporate three key elements:

1. *realizing* the prevalence of trauma;
2. *recognizing* how trauma affects all individuals involved with the program, organization, or system, including its own workforce; and,
3. *responding* by putting this knowledge into practice" [30].

Again, definitions of the basic principles underlying trauma-informed care vary in the literature but are relatively similar. The five values of care set out by Dr. Stephanie Covington, Center for Gender and Justice, comprise:

1. Safety: ensuring that women seeking services feel physically and emotionally safe.
2. Trustworthiness: women know that providers and practitioners will ensure that expectations are clear and consistent and that appropriate boundaries (especially interpersonal ones) are maintained.

3. Choice: preferences of the women seeking services in routine practices and crisis situations will be prioritised.
4. Collaboration: input from women will be considered in practices and decisions so that a collaborative relationship will be encouraged between those seeking services and service providers.
5. Empowerment: services are developed and delivered to maximise women's empowerment, recognising strengths and building skills [31].

2.3.4 A Universal *and* Targeted Approach

Maternity services should maximise opportunities to identify women's experiences of trauma and offer targeted support where appropriate to address the issues that have been disclosed. In the case of historic experiences of trauma, this may mean liaising with perinatal mental health services and Adult and Child and Adolescent Mental Health Services (CAMHS) so that a woman can access treatment, referring her to a specialist midwife, prioritising her for continuity of carer, referring her to appropriate Voluntary and Community Services (VCS), developing a care plan that is shared with and delivered against by all maternity services practitioners and ensuring a woman is offered enhanced post-natal support through Health Visiting Services.

However, just as a universal approach is taken with measures to ensure infection control, so maternity services should employ a universal trauma-informed approach to ensure that women who have not disclosed past experiences of trauma are not re-traumatised and are given the best possible care. A universal system-wide trauma-informed framework would also allow maternity services practitioners to respond in the moment and in emergency situations to women affected by trauma in the most effective way. Finally, a universal approach that improved the way in which care is delivered would benefit not just women affected by trauma but all women accessing maternity services.

2.3.5 Designing a Trauma-Informed Service

One of the most effective ways to understand how women with histories of trauma experience maternity services is to do a "walk-through" of those services and consider how women might respond to every aspect of the journey. For example, a walk-through might reveal that a woman in labour experiences difficulties finding labour ward or feels unsafe accessing it at night-time, particularly if she is on her own, compromising her feelings of safety. She might feel intimidated by unwelcoming or brusque reception staff. The birth environment may not help maximise women's feelings of safety or dignity. Asking service users with backgrounds of trauma to help with a walk-through and help share ideas about addressing the issues identified could be an effective way to begin learning how to improve those experiences.

The design of a trauma-informed framework and services should be collaborative and involve women with lived experience, maternity practitioners and other relevant stakeholders. Coproduction should be iterative, so that a system can continue to evolve and be improved. Continued input from service users should also be sought through maternity voices partnerships (MVPs) and public patient engagement (PPI) in partnership with other stakeholders working with trauma survivors including Voluntary and Community Services (VCS).

2.3.6 Understanding Prevalence and Early Identification of Issues

While we have some indications of the prevalence of trauma amongst women in the general population, maternity systems do not routinely record this data. In a recent study [25], women who had experienced trauma said they wanted midwives to ask them more about their situations at home, and not to assume that everything was fine. Early identification of issues and subsequent swift referrals were shown to maximise opportunities for women to access support.

2.3.7 Continuity of Care

Accessing continuity of care is of huge significance to women with experiences of trauma, enabling them to overcome their fear and distrust of services and develop trusted relationships, with midwives in particular, in which disclosure and the development of meaningful personalised care plans become much easier. Maternity services should prioritise continuity of care for women known to have experienced trauma or those known to be at higher risk of having a background of trauma, such as women who face multiple complex factors. But what about those who aren't identified, don't disclose or for whom continuity of care isn't an option? In a trauma-informed maternity system, women would experience continuity of care through a range of factors:

- Continuity of carer where possible.
- Universal understanding of trauma, enabling all practitioners to recognise and respond appropriately to signs of a trauma history wherever and whenever they were encountered.
- Continuity of culture, meaning that everyone a woman comes into contact with throughout her perinatal journey will treat her with respect, kindness and compassion regardless of her situation or perceived situation.
- Continuity of data, meaning that information about a woman's experiences and needs will be shared, with her consent, with all of her caregivers to ensure that she is not required to keep reiterating her past traumatic experiences.
- Continuity of approach, ensuring that women's wishes and choices are listened to and respected at every stage.

2.3.8   Choice and Consent

Women should be supported to create individualised care plans that reflect their needs, and these should be respected as far as possible. Where women have choices to make about their care, they should be informed by the evidence base and supported in a non-judgemental way by practitioners. Practitioners should not coerce or threaten women into making certain decisions – for example, into choosing or not choosing to give birth by elective caesarean section.

Meaningful consent should always be sought. Women who do not speak English should be helped to understand the procedures being recommended or decisions to be made through translation services where appropriate. Wherever possible, practitioners should take the time needed to explain a procedure and, when a woman has consented, to take the time to carry out the procedure at a pace that is comfortable for the woman. If a woman asks for a procedure to stop, it should stop [32].

2.3.9   Integrated Care

A whole systems approach will also involve working with other services outside maternity. For some women whose trauma lies in the past, albeit unresolved, mental health services will be key partners. Some women's experiences of trauma will also inform their situations and the services with which they are in contact with in the present. Pregnancy, birth and motherhood may not be their most urgent considerations, secondary to homelessness or inadequate housing; involvement with social services and the prospect their baby may be removed; a hostile immigration environment; domestic violence and abuse. As a result of these situations, women may also be in contact with other statutory bodies such as Children's Social Services, drug and alcohol services and/or voluntary and community services (VCS).

Maternity services should work holistically with the other stakeholders involved in women's lives, and being trauma informed will facilitate this woman-centred approach. Maternity services should be aware of the value of the VCS in providing care for women that is complimentary to statutory services. For example, the charity Birth Companions delivers targeted antenatal classes for women with very complex social needs in Hackney, London. The programme is funded by the area's Clinical Commissioning Group, and Birth Companions works closely with midwives at the Homerton Hospital who refer women.

2.3.10   Care of Staff

Taking good care of staff, and recognising the part that trauma plays in their lives and professional practice, should be an integral part of a trauma-informed maternity system. Support structures such as reflective practice and therapeutic supervision should be considered. Staff should be given the training and support to understand the impact of trauma on their professional practices and how that informs the care that they give women. This may incorporate their own lifetime trauma experiences as well as birth-related trauma. Trauma-informed practices could hold potential to improve the experiences and retention of staff.

2.3.11 Implementing Trauma-Informed Practice in Maternity Services

NHS England's recently published guide *A good practice guide to support implementation of trauma informed support in the perinatal period* provides further guidance [33].

2.4 Conclusion

This chapter demonstrated how childhood, adult and gendered experiences of trauma impacted adversely on the experiences and outcomes of women during pregnancy, birth and the postpartum period, examined existing trauma-related practice in maternal health and looked at the case for the introduction of a trauma-informed approach within maternity services. Limitations include the lack of evidence on the impact of trauma-informed care of pregnant women and new mothers, particularly across whole maternity systems (as no such practice currently exists).

Recommendations:
- Further research is needed on the impact of a trauma-informed approach in the care of pregnant women and new mothers.
- The implementation of a trauma-informed approach across a maternity system should be supported and evaluated.
- New guidance recently published by NHS England/Improvement to support the implementation of trauma-informed care in the perinatal period in maternity and mental health services is a useful further resource.

Trauma and its Impact on the Perinatal Woman: Key Learning Points
- **At least 5% of childbearing women in England and Wales experienced extensive physical or sexual violence during childhood.**
- **6% of women in England and Wales experienced four types of abuse in childhood; 14% of women experienced three types of abuse in childhood [9].**
- **More than one in ten women (11%) were sexually assaulted during childhood [9].**
- **Lifetime trauma history, particularly trauma experienced in childhood, is linked with adverse or risk of adverse reproductive outcomes.**
- **A high prevalence of lifetime trauma history is evident in populations experiencing adverse reproductive outcomes such as women whose babies are taken into care, women who are subject to repeat care**

proceedings, perinatal women in prison and women experiencing multiple disadvantage.
- Lifetime trauma history is associated with a range of obstetric risk factors and poor outcomes. Childhood experiences of trauma in particular augment the likelihood of low birth weight from perinatal anxiety and depression.
- Trauma increases the risk of lifetime and antenatal depression and anxiety, which are associated with a range of adverse psychiatric and biological outcomes for mothers and children.
- Women who have experienced trauma are at a greater risk of developing birth-related PTSD and find it harder to resolve successfully.
- Some women experiencing severe disadvantage with a high incidence of lifetime trauma history feel poorly served by maternity services.
- Women experiencing severe disadvantage with a high incidence of lifetime trauma have reported a lack of trust in services; yet almost all women eventually engage with maternity services (unlike other services that may be present in their lives).
- Women have confirmed the positive impact of continuity of care, a compassionate, non-judgemental and inclusive approach.
- Experiences of birth-related trauma are very common amongst midwives and contribute strongly to time taken off work and retention issues.

Trauma-Informed Maternity Services: Key Learning Points
Five values of care:
1. Safety
2. Trustworthiness
3. Choice
4. Collaboration
5. Empowerment.

Trauma-informed maternity services should:
- Be both universal and targeted
- Be designed collaboratively with stakeholders including women with lived experience
- Identify trauma issues as early as possible
- Prioritise continuity of care for trauma survivors
- Practice continuity of care across the maternity system
- Facilitate meaningful choice and consent
- Work holistically with other services outside maternity systems including voluntary and community services (VCS)
- Find effective ways to support staff around trauma.

References

1. Winfrey O, Treating childhood trauma, CBS News. 2018. https://www.cbsnews.com/news/oprah-winfrey-treating-childhood-trauma/
2. Amara P. Pregnancy and birth can be dangerously traumatic for rape victims but I've found a way to help them, The Independent. 2016. https://www.independent.co.uk/voices/pregnancy-and-birth-can-be-dangerously-traumatic-for-rape-victims-but-ive-found-a-way-to-help-them-a7073976.html
3. Substance Abuse and Mental Health Services Administration. SAMHSA's working definition of trauma and principles and guidance for a trauma-informed approach. Rockville, MD: Substance Abuse and Mental Health Services Administration, 2012. p. 2.
4. Mersky JP, Topitzes J, Reynolds AJ. Impacts of adverse childhood experiences on health, mental health, and substance use in early adulthood: a cohort study of an urban, minority sample in the US. Child Abuse Negl. 2013;37(11):917–25.
5. Crouch E, Radcliff E, Strompolis M, Srivastav A. Safe, stable, and nurtured: protective factors against poor physical and mental health outcomes following exposure to adverse childhood experiences (ACEs). J Child Adolesc Trauma. 2019;12(2):165–73.
6. Hughes K, et al. The effect of multiple adverse childhood experiences on health: a systematic review and meta-analysis. Lancet Public Health. 2017;2:e356–66.
7. McEwen B. Allostasis and allostatic load: implications for neuropsychopharmacology. Neuropsychopharmacology. 2000;22:108–24.
8. Bellis MA, Hughes K, Leckenby N, Perkins C, Lowey H. National household survey of adverse childhood experiences and their relationship with resilience to health-harming behaviours in England. BMC Med. 2014;12:72.
9. Office for National Statistics, *Abuse during childhood: Findings from the Crime Survey for England and Wales, year ending March 2016*, The 2015 to 2016 Crime Survey for England and Wales. https://www.ons.gov.uk/peoplepopulationandcommunity/crimeandjustice/articles/abuseduringchildhood/findingsfromtheyearendingmarch2016crimesurveyforenglandandwales#things-you-need-to-know
10. Scott S and McManus, Hidden Hurt: Violence, abuse and disadvantage in the lives of women. 2016. DMSS Research for Agenda.
11. Adult Psychiatric Morbidity Survey: Survey of Mental Health and Wellbeing, England, 2014 (2016), NHS Digital. https://digital.nhs.uk/data-and-information/publications/statistical/adult-psychiatric-morbidity-survey/adult-psychiatric-morbidity-survey-survey-of-mental-health-and-wellbeing-england-2014
12. Putnam KT, Harris WH, Putnam FW. Synergistic childhood adversities and complex adult psychopathology. J Trauma Stress. 2013;26:435–42. https://doi.org/10.1002/jts.21833.
13. Cardwell V, and Wainwright L, *Making Better Births a reality for women with multiple disadvantages, a qualitative peer research study exploring perinatal women's experiences of care and services in north-east London* (Birth Companions/Revolving Doors 2018).
14. Montgomery E et al. The re-enactment of childhood sexual abuse in maternity care: a qualitative study, BMC Pregnancy and Childbirth. 2015.
15. Kennedy A et al. The Birth Charter for women in prisons in England and Wales, Birth Companions. 2016.
16. Onoye JM, Goebert D, Morland L, Matsu C, Wright T. PTSD and postpartum mental health in a sample of Caucasian, Asian, and Pacific islander women. Arch Women Ment Hlth. 2009;12:393–400. https://doi.org/10.1007/s00737-009-0087-0.
17. Onoye et al., 2009.
18. Rogal et al., 2007.
19. Blackmore ER, Putnam FW, Pressman EK, Rubinow DR, Putnam KT, Matthieu MM, Gilchrist MA, Jones I, O'Connor TG. The effects of trauma history and prenatal affective symptoms on obstetric outcomes. J Trauma Stress. 2016;29(3):245–52. https://www.ncbi.nlm.nih.gov/pmc/articles/PMC4902169/

20. Ayers S, Bond R, Bertullies S, Wijma K. The aetiology of post-traumatic stress following childbirth: a meta-analysis and theoretical framework. Psychol Med. 2016;46(6):1121–34. ISSN 1469-8978
21. www.birthtraumaassociation.org.uk
22. Sheen K, Spiby H, Slade P. Exposure to traumatic experiences of posttraumatic stress symptoms in midwives: prevalence and association with burnout. Int J Nurs Stud. 2015;52(2):578–87.
23. Sheen K, Spiby H, Slade P. The experience and impact of traumatic perinatal event experiences in midwives: a qualitative investigation. Int J Nurs Stud. 2016;53:61–72.
24. Broadhurst K, et al. Vulnerable mothers and recurrent care proceedings. Centre for Child & Family Justice Research/ Lancaster University; 2017.
25. Cardwell V et al, *Making Better Births a reality for women with multiple disadvantages*: A qualitative peer research study exploring perinatal women's experiences of care and services in north-east London, Revolving Doors. 2018.
26. Seng J et al. Trauma-informed care in the perinatal period, Dunedin. 2015.
27. Clewett, N and Pinfold, V; Evaluation of Birth Companions' Community Link Service, McPin Foundation (2015)
28. McPin.
29. Thomson, G and Balaam, M-C, Experiences and Birth Outcomes of Vulnerable Women, University of Central Lancashire (2016)
30. Substance Abuse and Mental Health Services Administration. SAMHSA's working definition of trauma and principles and guidance for a trauma-informed approach. Rockville, MD: Substance Abuse and Mental Health Services Administration; 2012. p. 4.
31. Covington S. Becoming trauma informed: tool kit for women's community service providers, Center for Gender and Justice.
32. For more comprehensive information about informed consent, refer to Birthrights factsheet found at https://www.birthrights.org.uk/factsheets/consenting-to-treatment/.
33. Law, C., et al. A good practice guide to support implementation of trauma informed care in the perinatal period; Blackpool Better Start Centre for Early Childhood Development (2021). https://www.england.nhs.uk/wp-content/uploads/2021/02/A-good-practice-guide-to-support-implementation-of-trauma-informed-care-in-the-perinatal-period-February-2021.pdf

Black Asian Minority Ethnic (BAME) Women's Experiences of Maternity Care

3

Tawanda Bvumburai

Abstract

The statistics show that there are major disparities when it comes to Black, Asian and Minority Ethnic (BAME) women in maternity. Black women are five times more likely to die, and Asian women are twice as likely to die than their White counterparts. Babies that are born to BAME women also have the highest infant mortality rate in the UK.

The history of racism and the evolution of racism plays a key part on the disparities. An audit of Black, Asian and Ethnic Minority women were asked about their experiences of maternity care, along with midwives who care for BAME women. The results reflect the emerging evidence from research and reports.

Unconscious bias and conscious bias play a substantial role in the care BAME women are given. There needs to be a national drive for training, and policies need to be created to mitigate the mortality and morbidity rate for BAME women and their babies.

Keywords

Unconscious bias · Black, Asian and Minority Ethnic (BAME) · Women · Racism · Pain

Key Learning Points

By the end of this chapter, you will:

- Know key statistics and research about BAME women's experience of maternity care.

T. Bvumburai (✉)
Complex social care and FGM specialist Midwife, Hatfield, UK

© Springer Nature Switzerland AG 2021
L. Abbott (ed.), *Complex Social Issues and the Perinatal Woman*,
https://doi.org/10.1007/978-3-030-58085-8_3

- Have an insight into the history of racism and how this can impact BAME women's care.
- Have an understanding of lived experiences.
- Understand how unconscious bias affects BAME women and the healthcare system as a whole.

3.1 Introduction

This chapter explores issues in relation to the experiences of BAME women in maternity. The research evidence and historical context of racism in maternity services and healthcare in general will be described. Some of the myths relating to perceptions of Black women's experiences of pain will be discussed. Drawing upon current reports, this chapter reflects on why Black women are five times and Asian women twice more likely to die. The words of Black women and midwives illuminate experiences of racial bias. It essential to understand why BAME women have poorer, traumatising and fatal experiences within maternity. This chapter will also explore themes that contribute to the outcomes in maternity care for BAME women.

3.2 Statistics and Evidence from National Studies

The office of national statistics (2017) reports that just over a quarter of the women that give birth in England are of an ethnic minority [1].

According to the 2020 Mothers and Babies: Reducing Risk through Audits and Confidential Enquiries across the UK (MBRRACE-UK) report [2, 3], Black women are 5 times more likely and Asian women twice as likely to die from childbirth and pregnancy-related issues in comparison to their White counterparts.

Knight et al. (2019) identify that although Black and Asian women only make up 14% of women giving birth, they make up 34% of women that die [2]. Specifically, Black women only make up 4% of women that give birth but 18% of women that die. The Office for National Statistics (ONS) in 2015 also reports that babies from ethnic minority women have the highest infant mortality rate, e.g. Pakistani babies = 6.7, Black Caribbean babies = 6.6 and Black African babies = 6.3 deaths per 1000 live births [4].

Henderson, Gao and Redshaw (2013) [5] found that ethnic minority women had poorer experiences of maternity care than White women, and a systematic review exploring ethnic minorities [6] found that the themes of issues around healthcare services and systems, culture and social needs, communication and midwife-woman relationship were constant for women from ethnic minority backgrounds.

3.3 History of Racism in Healthcare Settings

BAME women's experiences are shaped by history and the behaviours perpetrated over time. The overtness of racism may have changed; however, the subtle behaviours are equally harmful to BAME women. It is important to understand what is currently happening, in order to understand why Black women are five times and Asian women two times more likely to die than their White counterparts in this current day. History shows that this is when fundamental practices, discrimination and bias were originally engraved into healthcare. A historical context enables us to have a helicopter view on why there may be poorer outcomes for BAME women. We must also recognise that there is a horrific, brutal and heart-wrenching history of racism and crimes against ethnic groups from slavery and colonialism days. Although slavery was abolished and the countries were decolonised, we must recognise that the world has spent more time in this type of regime than the time that we have been out of it. Therefore, it is not surprising that there is lasting dominance of the minds, processes, laws and conduct of the oppressors and their generational offspring. It must also be recognised that the lasting trauma and effects on ethnic groups from these times take centuries to heal and recover from. However, there is hope that by recognising these misfortunes, there can be real change of outcomes of BAME women in maternity care for the better.

There is limited research undertaken in the UK with regard to racial inequalities in healthcare. It has been highlighted in the last 15 years and most recently in the wake of the 2020 MBRRACE [3] report, combined with the Black Lives Matter movement that a lot of 'untold' history has surfaced. In this instance, untold means not taught in mainstream education and therefore may perpetuate false narratives and minimise the severity of racist history in healthcare settings.

3.3.1 Perceptions of how BAME Women Experience Pain: Myths Perpetuated Unconscious Bias

The perception of how BAME women perceive pain is one of the reasons why they are more likely to die from childbirth and pregnancy-related conditions. A notion was created by respected medical professionals and has been woven through healthcare for years. The potential for perpetuating myths means that the unconscious racism and bias taught in healthcare impact upon the mortality and morbidity rates for BAME women.

Dr. James Marion Sims was an American surgeon who was known as the 'father of modern gynaecology' [7]. He invented the vaginal speculum and pioneered a surgical technique to repair vesicovaginal fistula. Both are still important, used and performed today in obstetrics and gynaecology by doctors, midwives and nurses. However, what is not taught is that it is reported that Sims used enslaved women to perform clinical experiments without pain relief as he operated from the racist notion that 'Black women do not feel pain'. Furthermore, with Sims being such an influential figure in medical history, this notion has been held throughout healthcare worldwide.

Knight (2009) found that severe maternal morbidities were significantly higher in Black African, Black Caribbean and Pakistani women than for White women [8]. The statistics were also very similar when it came to maternal death rates. They initially believed it may be due to pre-existing medical conditions or care in pregnancy and/or labour. It could be said that this is simply not good enough and both BAME and White women have been giving birth since time immemorial. Therefore, there is no racial group that should be at a higher risk of negative outcomes. However, the racial inequalities that happen globally in all sectors could be the answer as to why this is happening.

Healthcare workers are still participants in the world and are part of the racial bias, prejudice and discrimination that happen outside of medicine. It would be almost impossible for us to assume that this turns off when they assume their healthcare role.

Hoffman (2016) undertook a study on racial bias in pain assessment and treatment recommendations, combined with untrue beliefs about biological differences between Black and White people [9]. Being a recent study, it demonstrates that false beliefs and practices may have been woven through time and consequently have detrimental current significance for BAME women in maternity [9]. Hoffman et al (2016) found that White adults without medical training believed there were biological differences in pain perception between Black and White people. It is well documented that there are discrepancies in pain management between the two groups and important that we understand the correlation between these beliefs that contribute to racial bias and the reasons why it is important. The second study by Hoffman et al. (2016) [9] found that there was a 'white fragility' in the perception of pain, and therefore, the racial bias meant that the 'Black strength' with regard to managing pain meant that there were differences in pain management by healthcare professionals.

Furthermore, there are books published as recent as 2014–2017 that support historical racist notions, with perceptions of pain in different cultures. Byrne's (2010) [10] *Nursing: A Concept-Based Approach to Learning*, First Edition erroneously outlined cultural responses to pain. The publishers later apologised; however, this information has already been used as a learning tool and therefore potentially learnt and absorbed by healthcare professionals internationally, potentially adversely affecting the care of BAME women.

3.3.1.1 Example of Bias in Textbook for HCPs

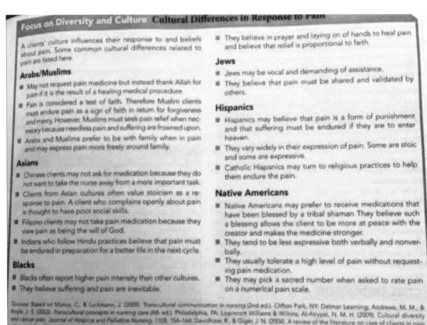

It is also paramount to understand the traumas associated with maternity and pregnancy (outlined in Naomi Delap's chapter discussing trauma-informed care). Although there are high rates of breastfeeding for BAME women, there is historical trauma in relation to slavery and colonialism. Enslaved women were often forced to breastfeed their slave masters' children as a form of labour. However, this meant that they were not able to feed their own children, due to the demand of female slave owners to feed their children. Often enslaved children were left to starve and die or taken by male slave owners to be used as alligator bait in order to make shoes and belts for themselves. The intent of slavery and colonialism was to gain by oppression, free labour, murder, torture, rape and a plethora of other tactics to gain control for the benefit of the White race. The lasting effects of this will take years to unlearn and to relearn nonracist/non-bias beliefs and behaviours. Whilst some of these unconscious behaviours are perpetuated onto BAME people as whole, there is also the conscious behaviours. The result of this means that the BAME community is underrepresented and mistreated throughout society; therefore, it is not a surprise that this spills into the care of BAME women in maternity.

After slavery was abolished, Black women were paid high wages to 'wet nurse'; however, this was likened to prostitution and was shunned. West and Knight (2017) [11] discussed the trauma enslaved women experience in relation to wet nursing and how this has had a generational effect on Black women and their maternity and breastfeeding experiences. West and Knight (2017) [11] report breastfeeding was associated with being poor and lowering down on the socio-economic scale; it could be said that this has shaped the current practices of breastfeeding in the world.

The pain BAME women have endured throughout history whilst still surviving has created a narrative of the 'strong Black woman'. The narrative may affect the person looking after Black women whilst also affecting the Black women. As explained above, healthcare workers throughout history have the notion that Black people perceive plain differently. Jerald et al. (2017) [12] found that Black women's awareness of other groups having negative stereotypes of them affects their health and well-being. BAME women tend to show pain in a less dramatic manner, as they believe they will be judged or cause annoyance if they are vocal, and this is partially because of the stereotypes created. Furthermore Rosenthal and Lobel (2016) [13] undertook a study and found that stereotypes affect the way Black women are treated whilst pregnant, and assumptions due to the stereotypes meant that Black women had poorer outcomes in maternity.

3.3.2 Midwives and BAME Women's Experiences in Maternity

As aforementioned, there are a significant amount of BAME women dying in maternity in comparison to their White counterparts [3]. Not only are BAME women being affected, but their babies also have a higher infant mortality rate.

These two statistics are intertwined with each other and need to be addressed for healthcare workers to understand, change behaviours and ultimately see the survival rate of BAME women and their babies rise. We must recognise the underlying health complications of BAME women. Research has shown that BAME women are more likely to suffer from gestational diabetes, pre-eclampsia and heart disease [14], and there is awareness of the trends and statistics of BAME women demonstrated through policies such as glucose tolerance tests for all BAME women between 24 and 28 weeks regardless of history. Therefore, it is important to reflect upon why BAME women are still more likely to die, support campaigns such as FIVEXMORE and respond to findings of inquiries.[1,2] The following is an exploration of racism in the workplace through an audit of midwives and BAME women.

3.4 Experiences of Racism in the Workplace

Behaviours and beliefs outside of the healthcare environment may influence treatment of certain groups within the workplace. Essentially if you have racist thoughts, these cannot turn off once you start working and turn on once you leave. Racism will be woven into everything because of beliefs, probably perpetuated throughout family generations. Experiences of racism in the workplace are illuminated through an audit of BAME and White midwives from different hospitals. Questions were asked about their experiences of looking after BAME women in maternity. Psuedonyms are used to anonymise health trusts, and midwives and responses are summarised verbatim.

My experiences of looking after BAME women in maternity include things such as discrimination towards the women, lack of understanding for cultural differences and lack of information given to these women compared to their white British counterparts. It can be difficult addressing these with your colleagues as people don't want to discuss such topics and for their downfalls to be highlighted as practitioners who believe that treat all women fairly, but they don't. Some of them have unconscious bias which shows in the level of care BAME women receive. (**Black midwife from Sunshine Trust**)

---

[1] https://www.birthrights.org.uk/2021/02/07/new-inquiry-to-drive-action-on-racial-injustice-in-maternity-care/

[2] https://www.fivexmore.com/

I have witnessed first-hand, derogatory and disgraceful comments by colleagues, which is frankly astonishing. Just last week, the midwife that handed over to me, decided to comment that and I quote "Just so you know this woman's partner is Black". I was shocked to hear this. I challenged the midwife and asked her to explain what she meant by such a comment and why did she feel it was imperative to tell me such a thing? She seemed shocked by my response, and this was followed by an apology. What concerns me more so, is this midwife, felt comfortable in speaking such things with me, who knows maybe because I appear white? But what is more alarming, is what is going through people's minds who care for BAME women and families... this is where the challenge lays, the ones who present open minded but harbour deep thoughts of inequality and bias that are systematic, whether conscious or unconscious. This for me is a challenge. **(White Midwife, Sunshine Trust)**

I don't think I've outwardly witnessed racism, but I definitely feel a lack of effort in people's care towards BAME women, especially when there's a language barrier involved. I also don't think there's enough chance for people to speak up on racial bias but maybe as a white woman, I'm not being offered the chance.

I think it's harder to get a doctor to listen to your concerns when it involves a BAME woman. Especially when we know that a lot of conditions in pregnancy affect BAME women more than others. I don't feel as if they get all the information sometimes and are able to make informed choices. A lot of their requests are ignored and not listened to with their birthing choices. They get the stigma of being the 'angry Black woman' or if it's an Indian woman I've had a lot of doctors call them a 'princess' and things like that. I find the same with the partners, if they are of a BAME group as well, the women are treated differently too. **(White Midwife, Rainbow Trust)**

Midwives from different trusts and from different races have demonstrated that they have witnessed the neglect of BAME women in maternity and their experiences. This supports the research undertaken so far on the BAME woman's experience in maternity [6]. Garcia et al. (2015) [14] found that although BAME women have access to services, they felt that they were not treated as individuals. There are certain barriers and facilitators that prevent BAME women from using maternity services. Garcia et al. (2015) [14] also report that the research that has undertaken does not promote a culturally competent maternity service. Therefore, there needs to be a national policy level that promotes a culturally competent service rather than just supplementary.

BAME women that have used maternity services in England were audited about their retrospective experiences of maternity care. What follows are summaries of verbatim responses from women to illuminate their past experiences.

When I was on the postnatal ward. The HCAs would not offer me drinks although they would ask and give all the other women in the bay. They would come and ask me later when the tea or coffee was cold. The Midwives advised all the other white women in the bay, that they would be showing them how to wash their babies for when they got home, however while they were in the hospital the midwife would wash their babies. I wasn't aware of this, and so when I saw everybody gathering, I didn't know what was happening, I was then asked, almost like an add on if I would like to see. The Midwives would wash all the other babies and leave my baby and so I just got on with it and washed my baby myself. They would also take all the other babies to the nursery at night, so the mums could get sleep, but they would never take mine. **(BAME woman who gave birth in the 1980s)**

I went into the hospital with really bad tummy pain, I knew something was not right. When I arrived in the hospital, they told me to sit and wait and I was in so much pain, I was crying. I kept going to the desk to tell them and they said I need to wait my turn. After 45mins, I said that I was bleeding and all the blood was all over the chair, they rushed me to a monitor and could find my baby's heartbeat. They rushed me to do a c-section and my son was born. My son was born with brain damage and had to stay in the special care unit for 6 weeks after he was born. They told me my placenta had abrupted and that why I was bleeding. I just feel they ignored me and the pain I was in. I couldn't see anybody else waiting, so I didn't understand why they just made me wait for so long even though they could see I was in pain. I have been caring for my son for 20 years and he will never be independent, I love him so much, however I often wonder what would have happened if they had seen to me earlier. The hospital was sued and we did receive a pay-out but no money will ever make reverse my sons brain damage. **(BAME woman in 2000)**

I had a C-section because my baby pooed in my womb. I came out of theatre and it was around four hours after my surgery that the midwives had changed shifts and a new midwife started looking after me. As soon as she came into my bay, she said "come on, you need to get up, we are not going to look after your baby all night, you need to do it yourself". I was so upset because it was my first baby, I literally could not feel my legs and I was in pain. Later when I asked for pain relief, I was told I couldn't have the strong stuff because I don't look like I am in pain and it will take longer for me to be discharged. I had only had the C-section 10 hours previous and I just broke down into tears. The midwife was very dismissive, and I just felt like I was a burden. **(BAME Woman 2009)**

When I was having my first baby, I started having contractions, I waited until they were five minutes apart and I went into the hospital. The midwife that saw me, was so horrible. She was talking so loudly, like I didn't understand English. When she was asking me about what had been happening, she said that whilst I was having contractions, I didn't look like I was in much pain, so they are going to send me home, I need to come back when, I am having three contractions in 10 minutes. I was in excruciating pain, my waters broke, and I had to stay in. I just felt I wasn't listened to. **(BAME woman)**

I had a good experience, all the midwives that looked after me were so kind. During the time I was in hospital, I had two black midwives and three white midwives. I felt very humbled by the way they looked after me. I felt they cared for me like I was their sister or their daughter. Nothing felt too much, I was feeling very vulnerable at the time and I lost all my dignity, but I was made to feel really comfortable. **(BAME Woman 2015)**

From the small sample of BAME women audited, it appears they are experiencing disparities at an increasingly higher rate. The experiences expressed above are further supported by Henderson et al. (2013) [5] and Jomeen and Reshaw (2012) [15] who found that there were poor staff attitudes and stereotyping in relation to BAME women's care. It was also found that healthcare staff took longer to respond to BAME women's needs which meant that there were longer hospital stays on the postnatal ward.

Pause for Personal Reflection
- Write down three words you felt when reading the experiences of women and midwives.
- Please reflect upon any workplace experiences where a woman's race or cultural background was discussed in relation to her response to pain. How did this make you feel?

3.4.1 BAME Women's Experiences Need to Improve

The Office of Diversity and outreach (2020) [16] define *unconscious bias* as social stereotypes about certain groups of people that individuals form outside their own conscious awareness. Everyone holds unconscious beliefs about various social and identity groups, and these biases stem from one's tendency to organize social worlds by categorizing [16]. Marcelin et al. (2017) found that unconscious bias can affect healthcare professionals in numerous ways that include hiring and promotion, patient and clinician interaction and inter-professional communication and relationships.

The recognition and need to change behaviour are necessary and urgent, and reflections and recommendations need to be evaluated. Training programmes have been constructed in different parts of the world; it would be necessary for study to be done to assess the statistics to see this type of training is effective. Diversity creates a broadening of perspective and also gives insight into other ethnicities and groups for the entire workforce and service users. We live in a diverse society, and there are so many things that one cannot learn alone but only with the interaction from people in all diverse groups. An example of this would be if somebody in England has malaria, it is seen a life-threatening tropical disease, and this could evoke panic and may need a specialist to come and see the patient. However, in countries where malaria is prevalent, the healthcare professional there will have a good and successful insight of how to fight malaria in the most efficient and effective way. We have to understand that this will be a complicated and continuous effort from all healthcare professionals because of the difficulties in identifying these behaviours unless it is overt. We also have to recognise that when entering healthcare, you have duty of care that all service users are treated in a safe and respectful manner, and therefore, this needs to be a compulsory part of that [17]. In order for things to change, there needs to be a cooperative and collaborative effort from the diverse mix of healthcare professionals that are all working hard to make healthcare fair and accessible to all on a global level, free of bias, prejudice and discrimination. Whilst training is commencing, there needs to be policies created simultaneously that battle the disparities happening to BAME women in maternity. It is important to recognise that change cannot be effectively achieved without the efforts of all. It is evident that there is a disturbing history, in relation to racism and the healthcare system. Perinatal women dying because of institutional and individual racism and discrimination must stop. The extensive history of racism means that it has been embedded in several institutions such as education, healthcare and the justice system. The subtle, soft undertone racism can also be as harmful as the overt racism. There is optimism on the horizon. Courageous campaigns such as FIVEXMORE (See footnote 2) are calling to act on such disparities and hope to explore why Black women are five times more likely to die than their White counterparts. The charity group Birthrights (See footnote 1) has launched a national inquiry led by women with lived experiences alongside legal, maternity and racism experts. This inquiry will look specifically into maternity care and racial injustice in response to the failure to 'safeguard Black and Brown people's basic rights in childbirth'. Upon looking at the history and understanding how and where the current beliefs and practices come from, it is going to be challenging to change the system. Having said that, this does not mean that it should not be changed; in fact, it is paramount that it should.

3.5   Conclusion

This chapter has explored the statistics, research and history involved in BAME women's experiences of maternity care. The chapter drew upon the voices of women and midwives through an audit of their experiences of perceptions of racism women. It has highlighted the history, lived experiences and some professional recommendations of what can be done in the future to tackle disparities. There is a momentum for positive change in response to the reports and responses from BAME women. This chapter further adds evidence to campaigns and inquiries such as FIVEXMORE and Birthrights, illuminated through the experiences of BAME women and midwives and written in the hope that it will evoke positive change and help consistently bring positive outcomes.

References

1. *Births By Parents' Country Of Birth, England And Wales—Office For National Statistics.* [online] Ons.gov.uk. 2019. https://www.ons.gov.uk/peoplepopulationandcommunity/births-deathsandmarriages/livebirths/bulletins/parentscountryofbirthenglandandwales/2017#the-percentage-of-births-to-women-born-outside-the-uk-varies-considerably-between-areas [Accessed 7 November 2020].
2. Knight M, Bunch K, Tuffnell D, Shakespeare J, Kotnis R, Kenyon S, & Kurinczuk JJ (Eds.). *Saving lives, improving mothers' care: lessons learned to inform maternity care from the UK and Ireland confidential enquiries into maternal deaths and morbidity 2015-17.* https://www.npeu.ox.ac.uk/downloads/files/mbrrace-uk/reports/MBRRACE-UK%20Maternal%20Report%202019%20-%20WEB%20VERSION.pdf, 2019.
3. Knight M, Bunch K, Tuffnell D, Shakespeare J, Kotnis R, Kenyon S, Kurinczuk JJ, on behalf of MBRRACE-UK. Saving lives, improving mothers' care—lessons learned to inform maternity care from the UK and Ireland confidential enquiries into maternal deaths and morbidity 2016-18. Oxford: National Perinatal Epidemiology Unit, University of Oxford; 2020.
4. *Pregnancy and ethnic factors influencing births and infant mortality—Office For National Statistics.* Ons.gov.uk. 2015 https://www.ons.gov.uk/peoplepopulationandcommunity/healthandsocialcare/causesofdeath/bulletins/pregnancyandethnicfactorsinfluencingbirthsandinfantmortality/2015-10-14#cause-of-death-groups-by-gestational-age-and-combined-ethinc-group [Accessed 7 November 2020].
5. Henderson J, Gao H, Redshaw M. Experiencing maternity care: the care received and perceptions of women from different ethnic groups. BMC Pregnancy Childbirth. 2013;13:1.
6. Khan Z. Ethnic health inequalities in the UK's maternity services: a systematic literature review. Br J Midwifery., 2021. 2020;29:2.
7. Ojanuga D. The medical ethics of the 'father of gynaecology', Dr J Marion Sims. J Med Ethics. 1993;19(1):28–31. [Internet]. [cited 15 December 2020] https://www.ncbi.nlm.nih.gov/pmc/articles/PMC1376165/

8. Knight M, Kurinczuk J, Spark P, Brocklehurst P. Inequalities in maternal health: national cohort study of ethnic variation in severe maternal morbidities. BMJ. 2009;338:b542. [Internet] [cited 17 November 2020] https://www.bmj.com/content/338/bmj.b542.full.pdf+html.
9. Hoffman K, Trawalter S, Axt J, Oliver M. Racial bias in pain assessment and treatment recommendations, and false beliefs about biological differences between blacks and whites. Proc Natl Acad Sci. 2016;113(16):4296–301. [cited 9 November 2020] [Internet] https://www.ncbi.nlm.nih.gov/pmc/articles/PMC4843483/
10. Byrne M, Callahan B, Carlson K, Daley L, Margorian K, Phillips P, et al. Nursing: a concept based approach to learning. 2nd ed. Upper Saddle River, N.J: Prentice Hall; 2010.
11. West E, Knight R. Mothers' Milk: slavery, wet-nursing, and black and white women in the antebellum south. J South Hist. 2017;83(1):37–68. [cited 18 November 2020]; [Internet] https://muse.jhu.edu/article/647289/summary
12. Jerald M, Cole E, Ward L, Avery L. Controlling images: how awareness of group stereotypes affects Black women's well-being. J Couns Psychol. 2017;64(5):487–99. [cited 18 November 2020] [Internet] https://psycnet.apa.org/doiLanding?doi=10.1037%2Fcou0000233
13. Rosenthal L, Lobel M. Stereotypes of Black American Women related to sexuality and motherhood. Psychol Women Q. 2016;40(3):414–27. [cited 18 November 2020] [Internet] https://www.ncbi.nlm.nih.gov/pmc/articles/PMC5096656/
14. Garcia R, Ali N, Papadopoulos C, Randhawa G. Specific antenatal interventions for black, Asian and Minority Ethnic (BAME) pregnant women at high risk of poor birth outcomes in the United Kingdom: a scoping review. BMC Pregnancy Childbirth. 2015;15:1. [cited 21 November 2020] [Internet] https://link.springer.com/article/10.1186/s12884-015-0657-2#citeas
15. Jomeen J, Redshaw M. Ethnic minority women's experience of maternity services in England. Ethn Health. 2012;18(3):280–96. [cited 28 November 2020] [Internet] https://www.tandfonline.com/doi/abs/10.1080/13557858.2012.730608?src=recsys&journalCode=ceth20
16. The Office of Diversity and Outreach (2020) Unconscious Bias | diversity.ucsf.edu [Internet]. Diversity.ucsf.edu. 2020 [cited 29 November 2020]. https://diversity.ucsf.edu/resources/unconscious-bias#:~:text=Unconscious%20biases%20are%20social%20stereotypes,organize%20social%20worlds%20by%20categorizing.
17. Nursing and Midwifery Council. Midwives rules and standards 2019. London: NMC; 2019.

Balancing Risk and Need: Substance Misuse and Perinatal Women

4

Karen Mills

Abstract

The long-term health and development of babies and children are influenced by the factors which affect them during pregnancy and in the first months of life. This chapter explores the extent to which parental substance misuse is an issue which might compromise development. Starting with an exploration of findings from Serious Case Reviews, the chapter examines the evidence of risk. It argues that assessment needs to be refined by a better understanding of risk and a cognisance of the way in which multiple factors (substance misuse combining with mental ill health or domestic abuse) serve to heighten that risk. The chapter balances this with consideration of the strengths women have and the protective factors in families which act to reduce harms.

The chapter considers the role which midwives hold, as part of a multi-agency team, in safeguarding and promoting children's life chances. In doing so, it focuses on the ways in which building strong professional relationships with women can facilitate change. The chapter concludes that in a context where services offered to women who use drugs are often stigmatised and othering, the provision of care through the universal service of midwifery can be pivotal in the lives of women.

Keywords

Drug use · Safeguarding · Serious case review · Stigma · Risk assessment

K. Mills (✉)
University of Hertfordshire, Hatfield, Herts, UK
e-mail: k.mills@herts.ac.uk

© Springer Nature Switzerland AG 2021
L. Abbott (ed.), *Complex Social Issues and the Perinatal Woman*,
https://doi.org/10.1007/978-3-030-58085-8_4

Key Learning Points
This chapter will enable readers to:

- Consider the relationship between substance misuse and risk in parenting.
- Consider the triangulation of risk, need and strength in women who are or are about to become parents.
- Consider the benefits and pitfalls of multi-agency practice.
- Consider interventions for women in the context of midwifery and other universal services.

4.1   Introduction

Pregnancy and the first year of life are one of the most important stages in the life cycle. It is the point at which the foundation of future health, development and well-being are laid down. The long term outcomes for children are strongly influenced by the factors that operate during pregnancy and the immediate postnatal period. It is therefore imperative to ensure that babies in utero and the early stages of their lives receive the best possible care and that any vulnerabilities are recognised early and addressed quickly. This requires good quality multi-agency pre-birth or at birth assessments to be undertaken. (extract from Serious Case Review: 'Ben' (1))

Used to alter mood and perception, drugs are widely available in UK society. They are consumed to alter bodily systems for a medical purpose and extend into social and recreational circumstances [2, 3]. 'Drug use' is a common phenomenon which includes aspirin and chocolate as well as alcohol and illegal drugs [2]. Problematic drug use is somewhat different related to both health and social problems [4]. There are a range of theories of problematic use: moral, biological, social and psychological [5]. These combine, so that poverty, personal trauma and social learning need to be addressed collectively in responding to individuals' needs. The nature of problematic drug use is such that it dominates the lives of users, occluding the focus on other things. Drug use crowds out employment, relationships and family to become the prime focus of a person's life. Inevitably, this has an impact on parenting capacity, and it is this aspect of the lives of drugs users that is the focus of this chapter.

Problematic drug users are marginalised and othered [6, 7] in policy and popular discourses [8, 9]. The activities of these drug users are perceived as very different from, rather than on a continuum with, drug use in the mainstream population. That othering affects the type and mechanisms of service delivery: influencing conversations between professionals and service users, skewing risk assessment and undermining interventions [10]. It also has an impact on the capacity and desire of parents to seek help for difficulties, meaning that issues often come to light only when concerns have escalated to the level of child protection, opportunities to support and safeguard children earlier in their lives having been missed [11].

Starting by examining the impact of illegal drug use upon children, this chapter looks at specific issues for pregnant and perinatal women. It balances risk and need and draws upon findings from Serious Case Reviews[1] to explore the factors which are especially pertinent for health and social care professionals [12].

Interventions for drug users are supported by a strong evidence base, and this informs the development of services and specifically the commissioning of services for women. The chapter will examine the unique ways in which universal, health-orientated services can contribute to responsive service delivery and how, by employing skills from social work, health and social care professionals can be instrumental in overcoming factors of stigma and improve outcomes for perinatal women and their children.

4.2   Risk: Messages from Serious Case Reviews

Most drug-using women are of childbearing age [13], and parental substance use affects the lives of large numbers of children in the UK. Research commissioned by the government indicates that over 45,000 children in England live with a female parent who uses opiates [14] and 200,000 live with a dependent drinker [15]. The impact of a childhood affected by parental substance misuse includes lower educational attainment, poorer economic prospects and higher likelihood of drug and alcohol problems in adult life. These effects and their consequences have been acknowledged for some time [16, 17] but continue to be overlooked or underappreciated by professionals.

In identifying risk issues as they apply specifically to infants, information from Serious Case Reviews is helpful. Serious Case Reviews are convened by local authorities following an incident of harm to or the death of a child where there are concerns about how organisations or professionals worked together in relation to safeguarding [12]. A recent triennial analysis of SCRs indicated that drug use is implicated in 47% of cases [18]. The NSPCC holds the repository of Serious Case Reviews, and an examination of these undertaken for this chapter indicates issues, borne out by the literature, which are particularly germane for midwifery services. Analysis of SCRs for this chapter, examining injury and death to children under 6 months, identified key aspects of these wider findings related to health and midwifery professionals and throw light on practice improvements.

There are a number of issues which compromise good antenatal care for this group. Drug use in women is closely associated with poverty [13], and women face practical problems of temporary or insecure housing, travel and transport difficulties which impinge on their planning and accessing of services [19]. Dealing with chaotic lives, women may be less well supported in pregnancy by

---

[1] Serious case reviews: There is a legal requirement, as defined in statutory Guidance, Working Together to Safeguard Children 2018, to undertake a serious case review when abuse or neglect of a child is known or suspected and

- either a child has died, or
- a child has been seriously harmed and there are concerns about how organisations or professionals worked together to safeguard the child.

partners and family. These practical issues are surrounded by a constellation of emotional difficulties. Women's emotional response to their circumstances is complex. They may feel guilty about the ways in which their drug use is compromising the health of their baby and simultaneously fearful and resentful of interference by professionals and the potential risk of the removal of their baby [20]. As a result, secrecy and concealment are common features in the lives of drug-misusing parents. All this can lead to avoidance of involvement and poor engagement with professionals. Drug-using women often book in late for maternity care [19, 21, 22]. Late booking in means that women do not benefit from accurate dating of their pregnancy and early screening, and lose out on the chance to build consistent relationships with midwifery services during their pregnancy [20]. For women whose general health is already compromised, this is a further risk factor and results in low-birth-weight babies and disproportionately high infant mortality [13]. Babies may be born addicted to, or withdrawing from, drugs and may be at a greater risk of sudden unexplained death. These are factors which need active management during women's maternity care as Serious Case Reviews indicate that missed appointments continue to be associated with subsequent serious harm to children [23–25]. Research points to the need for active personal contact to support attendance: using handwritten notes and text messages to facilitate engagement.

Government guidance [13, 21] points to the risk presented to infants from parents who practice co-bedding while the parent is under the influence of drugs. Serious Case Reviews highlight this as a significant risk of harm to babies and children [26]; and several point up cases where older children have died, and the risk has still been underappreciated [26]. These cases suggest that there is a need for clear and unambiguous advice to parents and that it is crucially important not to be falsely reassured by other indicators of good or improving care where co-sleeping is thought to be taking place [27].

In responding to the challenges raised by drug-using parents, repeated SCR investigations show that professionals give too much credence to the views of parents. Pregnant drug users may be extremely hard to reach:

> Families who have inhabited 'the system' for decades are evidence that the 'system' designed to support them to overcome difficulties has not worked well enough. They are likely to have developed strategies to cope with this that are challenging to work with constructively (23 p14).

As a consequence, they may deny or understate their drug use or may act to avoid support services where substance misuse will be uncovered. Injuries and deaths to children have occurred repeatedly where workers have been overly influenced by the plausible rationale for events offered by the parent and not stepped back to make an assessment which is centred on the safety of the child [23].

Even where risk is identified accurately, workers can be drawn into over-optimism for a parent [28], hoping for more change than is viable, or than is feasible within the timescale required for the health and wellbeing of children [26, 29]. Lord Laming in his report following the death of Victoria Climbié coined the concept of 'respectful uncertainty' [30] to encompass the requirement placed upon professionals to balance engagement and the aspiration for positive change with a scepticism about the potential for such changed based upon knowledge of past behaviour. This is an important consideration for health and social care professionals working in women's health or maternity departments. The 'paramountcy principle' which states that under English law the child's best interest and welfare is the first and paramount consideration [31] is potentially in conflict with woman-centred practice [32] and can create situations where risk is underestimated or where midwives are reluctant to challenge negative behaviours for fear of compromising engagement with health services [26]. Wiffin and Butler [1] provide an example from a specific SCR which is emblematic of this issue:

> The midwives did recognise that A was vulnerable, but her openness, her positive approach, determination and action to change her circumstances, along with her compliance with appointments, reassured the midwifery professionals that there were no current concerns. This was overly optimistic practice. There should have been a pre-birth assessment at this stage to consider the balance across the strengths, of which there were a number, with the risks, of which there were more. (1 p8)

Processes are in place to support professionals in working together to form rounded and holistic assessments of risk. SCRs indicate that these pose other challenges for midwifery and healthcare professionals. The Common Assessment Framework (CAF) originated from the reform agenda following the Climbié inquiry in 2003. By identifying a family's support needs and strengths, it is intended to provide a 'needs led, evidence based tool to promote uniformity, ensure appropriate early intervention, reduce referral rates to local authority children's services and lead to the emergence of a common language amongst child welfare professionals' [33]. SCRs indicate that the process has not properly included the views of midwives, health visitors and others dealing with perinatal substance using women. These show occasions where concerns are identified but not appropriately escalated or issues are raised but disregarded. This latter eventuality is made more likely by the fact that health and social work professionals do not appear to share the common language aspired to by the CAF. SCRs show occasions where midwives have reported concerns to social work professional, but the terminology used leads the social worker to consider these simply as professional 'contacts'. 'There was no common language and understanding between professionals as to what constitutes a referral, what is determined as a contact and how professionals should challenge any of these applications if they are not in agreement' (25 p 9).

Overall, Serious Case Reviews indicate that there are areas where health and midwifery services need to be more cognisant of risk to children and infants and more able to bring their assessment of risk to safeguarding services. In doing so, an accurate sense of the manifestations of risk is essential.

4.3   Parenting, Substance Use and Risk Assessment

If the majority of the population uses drugs in some way in their lives, then condemnation of drug-using parents and a perception of women who use drugs as inherently risky to their children cannot follow. Some more refined analysis of risk must be employed to determine those children who may be hurt or neglected as a result of their parent's self-absorption, negligence or violence. As Galvani says: 'Poor parenting is the determinant of harm to children, whatever the reasons for it' (34 p87).

D.W. Wınnicott coined the idea of a 'good enough parent' [35]. In essence, the term means an ordinary parent whose skills are sufficient to guarantee the health, safety and stability of their children. The majority of the 11.8 children and young people living in the UK are raised by just such 'good enough' parents [36]. This includes parents who drink or use drugs but who continue to offer a stable environment in which children can thrive. However, where substance use acts in conjunction with other issues, both complexity and risk accumulate. Sidebotham et al.'s analysis [18] of serious case reviews between 2011 and 2014 indicated that while 47% include drug or alcohol as a factor in serious harm to children, risk rises significantly where drug use co-exists with other problems. While poverty, housing issues or the physical illness of a parent may add complexity to parents' lives and instability to children's care, risk rises most significantly where families face issues of domestic violence or mental ill health [18]. In these circumstances, complexity in the lives of parents leads to instability and unpredictability in their care of their children. Impaired physical care can lead to neglect, while a lack of emotional support or appropriate boundary setting can cause emotional abuse [37].

Professionals assessing risk and its impact on individual children can look for manifestations of risk in three key areas: physical health, social engagement and emotional wellbeing. Of these, physical care is most clearly observable. Diverting family resources towards drugs and alcohol can mean a reduced spend on children's food and clothes with consequences for children's diet and hygiene. Ultimately, this leads to poor physical health and wellbeing and a higher risk of neglect [21]. Professionals providing both ante- and postnatal care can be alert to difficulties in the lives of vulnerable women which undermine the physical health and safety of babies. This may be poverty related to drug use which has an impact on material provision in the home. Professionals need to be aware of the physical conditions into which the baby will be discharged. Newborns cannot voice their own wishes of feelings, but their basic needs are for safety, warmth and food. Assessment of the home environment should include the level of hygiene, provision of food and the money available to provide adequate heating and clothing. There is also an overlap between physical provision and the emotional preparedness which underpins it. In discussing preparation for the arrival of the baby, is the mother realistic in her expectations, and is she making appropriate preparation for his or her care? [22].

Similarly, in older children, the literature indicates that family disorganisation can disrupt children's school attendance and access to leisure activities, both structured and unstructured with consequences not only for levels of educational attainment [38] but also for social isolation and social development. In babies, this educational stimulation must be provided in the home and by the parent [24]. Midwives and healthcare professionals should ask themselves if the home is impoverished and if the parent is realistic about their new role or if they underestimate the needs of a newborn and the way in which the life of the adult must be reconfigured in response to that need.

Parenting style can be affected by drug use, with parents acting either negligently, overly authoritarian or overly emotional depending upon the parent's cycle of drug acquisition, use and withdrawal. This inconsistency can lead to problems in the child's attachment. These contribute to low self-esteem and potentially poor mental or emotional health with long-term consequences in later life [34, 39]. So, in assessing risk, midwifery and health professionals should look for a combination of practical and emotional/psychological issues:

- Poor physical health.
- Lack of physical resources.
- Low levels of stimulation.
- Unrealistic concepts of parenting.
- Inconsistency in parenting style.

While Sidebotham [18] does identify the fact that drug and alcohol use is implicated in a high percentage of Serious Case Reviews, this is seldom the only factor, and it is the complexity of a family's struggles rather than drug use per se which precipitates risk. These complexities are most often manifest as a combination of drug use with domestic violence or mental ill health [40], and where this is the case, the risk to children is considerable [41]. In such circumstances, women may be perceived as isolated anxious or depressed as well as physically hurt. The confluence of substance use and domestic violence causes risk to increase exponentially, underlining the requirement for good multi-agency liaison outlined above.

4.4   Exploring Positive Factors

A balanced assessment requires professionals not only to identify and communicate risk but to balance that risk appropriately with the strengths in parents' lives. This involves identification of the relationship between risk and protection [13, 42]. Even in chaotic families, there can be influences, people and situations which insulate children from the physical and emotional impacts of drug use. Identifying and acting to strengthen and support these is as important as reducing risks.

'Although parental alcohol and/or drug use can have a number of impacts on children and families, it does not necessarily follow that **all** children will be adversely affected' (13 s51) Although drug use does compromise the physical well-being of babies both in utero and after birth, the investigation of Serious Case Reviews indicates that significant, avoidable harms, neglect and death rarely occur where drug use alone is a feature. It is drug use in combination with other issues which is problematic and complexity which presents greatest danger [18]. Between one quarter and one third of adult drug users are women, a proportion which has remained relatively constant in recent years [4, 43]. In 2018, 31% of adults in treatment were women [44, 45]. Historically research has identified significant barriers to women seeking of drug treatment [46]; these included social, structural and economic factors as well as a history of treatment services orientated around the needs of White men which compounded the traumas experienced by women and which often have precipitated their drug use in the first place [47]. Pregnancy itself has been shown to be a complicating factor, and international research has observed the fact that pregnancy can lead to treatment dropout and lower retention [48].

However, more recent statistics and research indicate a brighter picture, suggesting that women are beginning to seek treatment sooner in their drug-using career, stay longer in treatment and have better outcomes [49]. Women in the general population make use of health and mental health services, including preventative healthcare proportionately more than men [50]; as treatment services become more responsive, offering more flexible times, better outreach and women-only services, it is possible to capitalise on that worldview in order to support vulnerable women to access drugs services as part of their wider healthcare needs.

Where there is a relationship with a non-drug-using carer (another parent or a grandparent for example), this can offer significant protection to children. Stable carers can help meet a child's basic needs for food, clothing and shelter as well as offering support in times of crisis [51, 52]. In the long term, such support can provide a secure base for attachment when the birth parent's emotional capacity is compromised [42]. Equally, support can be afforded by structured engagement from outside the family, nurseries and schools, peer support and social activities. These offer structure and respite in a life which might otherwise be chaotic. In the case of infants, the physical and emotional support which can be offered to a vulnerable new mother from the father and extended family should include an assessment of whether these persons are themselves non-drug users and able to offer practical help. Professionals should ask if such help is available and, if not, what support the mother will need in order to provide good enough basic care. Adults from the immediate and extended family or support services are resources for the child and act as a network of support and physical and emotional care. Building this helps children grow and thrive physically and develop a sense of personal wellbeing.

4.5   Interventions and the Role of Universal Services

Drug treatment remains a stigmatised service, accessed by women who are marginalised in society. A compelling stereotype exists that women who continue to use drugs in pregnancy are failing to protect their unborn child, reneging on their responsibilities as mothers [53, 54] and becoming 'dangerous vessels' for their babies (54 p37). This stigmatisation and objectification of women are pernicious and long-standing; women are perceived as rational actors [55] and drugs use perceived as a 'disease of will' (56 p2). Stigma can be social (where society endorses and promulgates a stereotype) or a process of self-stigma where the women themselves endorse a negative self-view, with all the accompanying emotions of self-loathing [57]. However, pregnancy and birth are watershed moments in the lives of women and can be a catalyst for change and new starts [10, 58]. Engaging with this offers an opportunity to engage with women positively in relation to treatment and healthcare and also offers an opportunity for them to recover their 'spoiled identity' [59]. Maternity care provides an opportunity for healthcare professionals to meet and support women, partners and their families who might otherwise never or rarely access health services [60]. This analysis suggests that midwives can play a crucial part in assisting women in a process of 'transformation… as women attempt to move out of drug use and towards motherhood' [10] p985). In order to do so, it is important to offer services which do not compound social and self-stigma [21]. While research by Fonti indicated that midwives and midwifery services do not in general share a stigmatised view of drug-using pregnant women [61], this cannot be assumed as simply a feature of the role, and there is a need for ongoing training and personal reflection to avoid the accretion of prejudice [19].

4.6 Conclusion

Working with women who use drugs during pregnancy is fraught with contradictions. Drug use of itself compromises the health of children, but serious long-term risk is usually found only where chaotic drug use co-exists with other issues (poverty, mental ill health or violence). Drug-using women book in late for maternity services and avoid contact with health and other professionals while simultaneously pregnancy offers a chance for change and new beginnings. Professionals engaged in supporting women in this change need to engage in a relationship of trust; doing so requires empathy and respect in understanding a woman's subjective experience and genuineness and honesty in offering feedback about her situation [62, 63]. Yet Serious Case Reviews highlight the fact that too much trust in women's plausible explanations of the reasons for continuing drug use precipitates risk to children. The paramountcy principle underlines the fact that in every case the needs of the child must be prioritised over those of the mother. For services engaged to meet the needs of women at one of the most vulnerable times in their lives, this can be a difficult concept to adhere to.

In forming a holistic assessment, health professionals should examine the subjective circumstances of families in order to respond to risk as it is manifest in *this* woman at *this* time. Doing so requires active engagement with other professionals and transparent, honest conversations with women. There are structural challenges in this as stretched maternity services struggle to offer continuity of care; however, in the most complex cases, this is essential to support change and identify risk:

Building relationships is essential in safeguarding children and those relationships can only be built if there is continuity of input from at least one service provider. (64 p19)

In balancing of issues of risk with the aspiration for change, high-quality multi-agency practice is essential. Serious Case Reviews show that despite the aspiration of common working practices and common language, midwifery services have difficulty in having their voices and concerns heard. This is particularly important in light of the privileged position which practitioners in the discipline hold in in the lives of women. Workers intervene at a time of transition, and such transitions can trigger seismic change. Engaging with women and with other professionals in safeguarding services gives midwives the opportunity to effect real change.

References

1. Wiffin J & Butler V. *Serious case review: "Ben": overview.* Gloucestershire Local Safeguarding Children Board. 2016. Retrieved January, 17, 2019 from: https://library.nspcc.org.uk/HeritageScripts/Hapi.dll/retrieve2?SetID=BA5B6CF7-2704-41EB-8493-0320618D74F8&LabelText=Gloucestershire&SearchTerm0=%7E%5B%40GLOUCESTERSHIRE%5D%20%5E%20%25STA%20%5E%20%25EQU%20%5E%20%25EB%20%5E%20%25ENQ%7E&SearchPrecision=20&SortOrder=Y1&Offset=5&Direction=%2E&Dispfmt=F&Dispfmt_b=B27&Dispfmt_f=F13&DataSetName=LIVEDATA.
2. Gossop M. Living with drugs. Aldershot: Ashgate Publishing, Ltd.; 2013.
3. Rassool GH. *Alcohol and drug misuse: a handbook for students and health professionals*: Routledge. 2009.
4. EMCDDA. United Kingdom country drug report 2018. Drug use: prevalence and trends. Lisbon: EMCDDA; 2018. Retrieved January, 12, 2019 http://www.emcdda.europa.eu/countries/drug-reports/2018/united-kingdom/drug-use_en
5. Petersen T. *Working with substance misusers: a guide to theory and practice*: Routledge. 2005.
6. Jandt FE. Intercultural communication: a global reader. London: Sage; 2004.
7. Johnson JL, Bottorff JL, Browne AJ, Grewal S, Hilton BA, Clarke H. Othering and being othered in the context of health care services. Health Commun. 2004;16(2):255–71.
8. Goffman E. Notes on the management of spoiled identity. New Jersey: Prentice-Hall Englewood Cliffs; 1963.
9. Mills K. *Delivering drug treatment to new minority communities: fresh perspectives.* 2017. Retrieved 18th October 2019 from https://uhra.herts.ac.uk/bitstream/handle/2299/18188/02049013%20Mills%20Karen%20final%20submission.pdf?sequence=1&isAllowed=y.
10. Radcliffe P. Motherhood, pregnancy, and the negotiation of identity: the moral career of drug treatment. Soc Sci Med. 2011;72(6):984–91. https://doi.org/10.1016/j.socscimed.2011.01.017.
11. Public Health England. Problem parental drug and alcohol use: a toolkit for local authorities. London: Public Health England; 2018. Retrieved January, 15, 2019 from: https://www.gov.uk/government/publications/parental-alcohol-and-drug-use-understanding-the-problem
12. Department for Education. Working together to safeguard children a guide to inter-agency working to safeguard and promote the welfare of children. London: Stationery Office; 2018.
13. Scottish Government. *Getting our priorities right: good practice guidance. Updated good practice guidance for all agencies and practitioners working with children, young people and families affected by problematic alcohol and/or drug use.* Edinburgh: Scottish Executive; 2013. Retrieved January, 16, 2019 from https://www.gov.scot/publications/getting-priorities-right/pages/14/.
14. Hay G. *Estimates of the number of children who live with opiate users, England 2014/15.* Liverpool John Moores University/Public Health England. 2018 Retrieved January, 16, 2019 from: https://phi.ljmu.ac.uk/wp-content/uploads/2018/03/parental-report-March-2018-VH.pdf.

15. Public Health England. Innovation fund open to help children of dependent drinkers. London: Public Health England; 2018. Retrieved January 16, 2019 from: https://www.gov.uk/government/news/innovation-fund-open-to-help-children-of-dependent-drinkers
16. Kroll B, & Taylor A. *Parental substance misuse and child welfare*: Jessica Kingsley Publishers. 2003.
17. McKeganey N, Barnard M, McIntosh J. Paying the Price for their Parents' addiction: meeting the needs of the children of drug-using parents. Drugs: Educ Prev Polic. 2002;9(3):233–46. https://doi.org/10.1080/09687630210122508.
18. Sidebotham P, Brandon M, Bailey S, Belderson P, Dodsworth J, Garstang J, et al. Pathways to harm, pathways to protection: a triennial analysis of serious case reviews 2011 to 2014. London: Department for Education; 2016.
19. Radcliffe P. Substance-misusing women: stigma in the maternity setting. Br J Midwifery. 2011;19(8):497–506. https://doi.org/10.12968/bjom.2011.19.8.497.
20. Stephen G, Whitworth MK, Cox S. Substance misuse in pregnancy. Obstet Gynaecol Reprod Med. 2014;24(10):309–14. https://doi.org/10.1016/j.ogrm.2014.07.001.
21. ACMD. Hidden harm. London: Home Office; 2003. Retrieved from http://www.homeoffice.gov.uk/publications/agencies-public-bodies/acmd1/hidden-harm-full
22. Bedford A. Serious case review into services provided to Child S and Family. LSCB: Waltham Forest Safeguarding Children Board; 2017. Retrieved January, 17, 2019 from: https://library.nspcc.org.uk/HeritageScripts/Hapi.dll/search2?searchTerm0=C6692&_ga=2.4633907.1050319287.1534512297-790590817.1510157333
23. Carmi E & Peel S. *Serious case review: "Child J": overview*. Newcastle Safeguarding Children Board. 2016. Retrieved January, 17, 2019 from: https://www.nscb.org.uk/Serious%20Case%20Review.
24. Richardson L. Serious case review: Baby W and Child Z: overview. LSCB: Sunderland Safeguarding Children Board; 2016.
25. Richardson L & Grey J. *Serious case review: Baby E: overview*. Sunderland Safeguarding Children Board. 2016. Retrieved January, 17, 2019 from: https://library.nspcc.org.uk/HeritageScripts/Hapi.dll/retrieve2?SetID=B1CE61A2-7A4A-47D3-8D8F-F47E3E993EBD&LabelText=Sunderland&SearchTerm0=%7E%5B%40SUNDERLAND%5D%20%5E%20%25STA%20%5E%20%25EQU%20%5E%20%25EB%20%5E%20%25ENQ%7E&SearchPrecision=20&SortOrder=Y1&Offset=7&Direction=%2E&Dispfmt=F&Dispfmt_b=B27&Dispfmt_f=F13&DataSetName=LIVEDATA.
26. Pettitt N. *Serious case review: Child A: overview report*. Milton Keynes Safeguarding Children Board. 2016 Retrieved January, 17, 2019 from: https://library.nspcc.org.uk/HeritageScripts/Hapi.dll/retrieve2?SetID=60EE5AAE-E81F-4692-80CE-33D4FDC92A72&LabelText=Milton&SearchTerm0=%7E%5B%40MILTON%5D%20%5E%20%25STA%20%5E%20%25EQU%20%5E%20%25EB%20%5E%20%25ENQ%7E&SearchPrecision=20&SortOrder=Y1&Offset=3&Direction=%2E&Dispfmt=F&Dispfmt_b=B27&Dispfmt_f=F13&DataSetName=LIVEDATA
27. Davies H. *Serious case review: Child S*. Swindon Local Safeguarding Children Board. 2016 Retrieved January, 17, 2019 from: https://library.nspcc.org.uk/HeritageScripts/Hapi.dll/retrieve2?SetID=0F9E71C0-085F-4C4E-8B52-5E7293596F98&LabelText=Swindon&SearchTerm0=%7E%5B%40SWINDON%5D%20%5E%20%25STA%20%5E%20%25EQU%20%5E%20%25EB%20%5E%20%25ENQ%7E&SearchPrecision=20&SortOrder=Y1&Offset=2&Direction=%2E&Dispfmt=F&Dispfmt_b=B27&Dispfmt_f=F13&DataSetName=LIVEDATA
28. Dingwall R, Eekelaar J, Murray T. The protection of children: state intervention and family life. Oxford: Basil Blackwell; 1983.
29. Jones H. Report of learning together serious case review: Child M: presented to the Waltham Forest Safeguarding Children Board. Waltham Forest Safeguarding Children Board. 2017. Retrieved January, 17, 2019 from: https://library.nspcc.org.uk/HeritageScripts/Hapi.dll/retrieve2?SetID=EB6B5401-EBD5-44A8-AFD3-EED7F3047D1C&LabelText=Waltham&SearchTerm0=%7E%5B%40WALTHAM%5D%20

%5E%20%25STA%20%5E%20%25EQU%20%5E%20%25EB%20%5E%20%25ENQ%
7E&SearchPrecision=20&SortOrder=Y1&Offset=2&Direction=%2E&Dispfmt=F&Disp
fmt_b=B27&Dispfmt_f=F13&DataSetName=LIVEDATA

30. Laming H. The Victoria Climbié Inquiry. London: Department of Health and Home Office; 2003.
31. Children Act. 1989. Retrieved 18th October 2019 from: https://www.legislation.gov.uk/ukpga/1989/41/contents
32. Wainwright P, Gallagher A. Understanding general practitioners' conflicts of interests and the paramountcy principle in safeguarding children. J Med Ethics. 2010;36(5):302–5. https://doi.org/10.1136/jme.2009.034488.
33. Warren House Group, Dartington Social Research Unit. Towards a common language for children in need. Dartington: Dartington Social Research Unit; 2004.
34. Galvani S. Supporting people with alcohol and drug problems: making a difference. The Policy Press; 2012.
35. Winnicott D. The child, the family, and the outside world classics in child development. USA: Winnicott; 1957.
36. Cleaver H, & Unell I. *Children's needs-parenting capacity: child abuse, parental mental illness, learning disability, substance misuse, and domestic violence*: The Stationery Office. 2011.
37. NSPCC. *Parental substance misuse: how to support children living with parents who misuse alcohol and drugs*. 2018. Retrieved January, 17, 2019 from: https://www.nspcc.org.uk/preventing-abuse/child-protection-system/parental-substance-alcohol-drug-misuse/
38. Department for Education. The link between absence and attainment at KS2 and KS4. London: The Stationery Office; 2016.
39. Velleman R, Templeton L. Understanding and modifying the impact of parents' substance misuse on children. Adv Psychiatr Treat. 2007;13(2):79–89.
40. Middleton C, Hardy J. Vulnerability and the 'toxic trio': the role of health visiting. Community Pract. 2014;87(12):38.
41. Frederico M, Jackson A, Dwyer J. Child protection and cross-sector practice: an analysis of child death reviews to inform practice when multiple parental risk factors are present. Child Abuse Rev. 2014;23(2):104–15. https://doi.org/10.1002/car.2321.
42. Executive S. Getting our priorities right: good practice guidance for working with children and families affected by substance misuse. Edinburgh: Scottish Executive; 2003.
43. Best D, Abdulrahim D. Women in drug treatment services. Research briefing, 6. London: NTA; 2005.
44. National Statistics. Alcohol and drug treatment for adults: statistics summary 2017 to 2018. London: ONS; 2018. Retrieved January, 12, 2019 from: https://www.gov.uk/government/publications/substance-misuse-treatment-for-adults-statistics-2017-to-2018/alcohol-and-drug-treatment-for-adults-statistics-summary-2017-to-2018#parental-status-and-safeguarding-children
45. Public Health England. Adult substance misuse statistics from the National Drug Treatment Monitoring System (NDTMS). London: Public Health England; 2017. Retrieved January, 12, 2019 from: https://assets.publishing.service.gov.uk/government/uploads/system/uploads/attachment_data/file/658056/Adult-statistics-from-the-national-drug-treatment-monitoring-system-2016-2017.pdf
46. Greenfield SF, Brooks AJ, Gordon SM, Green CA, Kropp F, McHugh RK, et al. Substance abuse treatment entry, retention, and outcome in women: a review of the literature. Drug Alcohol Depend. 2007;86(1):1–21.
47. Becker J, Duffy C. Women drug users and drugs service provision: service-level responses to engagement and retention. London: Home Office; 2002.
48. Center for Substance Abuse Treatment. Substance abuse treatment for women. 2009.
49. National Treatment Agency. Women in drug treatment: what the latest figures reveal. London: NHS; 2010.

50. Thompson AE, Anisimowicz Y, Miedema B, Hogg W, Wodchis WP, Aubrey-Bassler K. The influence of gender and other patient characteristics on health care-seeking behaviour: a QUALICOPC study. BMC Fam Pract. 2016;17(1):38.
51. Barnard M. Between a rock and a hard place: the role of relatives in protecting children from the effects of parental drug problems. Child Fam Soc Work. 2003;8(4):291–9. https://doi.org/10.1046/j.1365-2206.2003.00297.x.
52. Ronel N, Haimoff-Ayali R. Risk and resilience: the family experience of adolescents with an addicted parent. Int J Offender Ther Comp Criminol. 2010;54(3):448–72. https://doi.org/10.1177/0306624x09332314.
53. Murphy S, & Rosenbaum M. *Pregnant women on drugs: combating stereotypes and stigma*: Rutgers University Press. 1999.
54. Stengel C. The risk of being 'too honest': drug use, stigma and pregnancy. Health Risk Soc. 2014;16(1):36–50. https://doi.org/10.1080/13698575.2013.868408.
55. O'Malley P, Huges G, McLaughlin E, & Muncie J. Drugs, risks and freedoms. *Crime prevention and community safety. New directions*. 2002. p. 279–296.
56. Valverde M. Diseases of the will: alcohol and the dilemmas of freedom. Cambridge University Press; 1998.
57. Livingston JD, Milne T, Fang ML, Amari E. The effectiveness of interventions for reducing stigma related to substance use disorders: a systematic review. Addiction. 2012;107(1):39–50.
58. McIntosh J, McKeganey N. Addicts' narratives of recovery from drug use: constructing a non-addict identity. Soc Sci Med. 2000;50(10):1501–10. https://doi.org/10.1016/S0277-9536(99)00409-8.
59. Goffman E. The presentation of self in everyday life. New York: Doubleday Anchor; 1959.
60. Department of Health. Maternity matters: choice, access and continuity of care in a safe service. London: Department of Health; 2007.
61. Fonti S, Davis D, Ferguson S. The attitudes of healthcare professionals towards women using illicit substances in pregnancy: a cross-sectional study. Women Birth. 2016;29(4):330–5. https://doi.org/10.1016/j.wombi.2016.01.001.
62. Coulshed V, Orme J, British Association of Social Work. Social work practice. 5th ed. Basingstoke: Palgrave Macmillan; 2012.
63. Forrester D, Kershaw S, Moss H, Hughes L. Communication skills in child protection: how do social workers talk to parents? Child Fam Soc Work. 2008;13(1):41–51. https://doi.org/10.1111/j.1365-2206.2007.00513.x.
64. Tudor K. Serious case review: Baby J. LSCB: Wiltshire Safeguarding Children Board; 2016.

Perinatal Mental Health Issues: Key Factors and Evidence Base for the Planning and Management of Care for Women Experiencing Generalised Anxiety Disorder

5

Jennifer Parker

Abstract

This chapter examines perinatal mental health and its impact, stigma, current midwifery practices and education and the influence of in vitro fertilisation (IVF) upon perinatal mental health and, in particular, antenatal anxiety. Looking at the current research and literature, it explores the effects of poor perinatal mental health and current practices and if these are sufficient. Midwifery education in perinatal mental health is scant; an improvement in this could lead to reduced stigma, better detection and, consequently, more women receiving treatment. At least 80,000 women a year in the United Kingdom suffer with generalised anxiety disorder, but the vast majority are either without effective treatment or in most circumstances undiagnosed, and this can lead to significant detriments to both the women and their babies' health. Providing routine mental health support to women could result in significant and vital savings.

Keywords

Generalised anxiety disorder · In vitro fertilisation · Midwifery · Stigma

5.1   Introduction

This chapter explores mental health issues paying specific attention to antenatal anxiety. The main focus being upon its impact on women and their families, stigma, support, treatment and midwives' education. The role of the midwife will be examined along with the evidence for the provision of maternity care. The chapter will

J. Parker (✉)
NHS, Hertfordshire, UK

© Springer Nature Switzerland AG 2021
L. Abbott (ed.), *Complex Social Issues and the Perinatal Woman*,
https://doi.org/10.1007/978-3-030-58085-8_5

focus upon the experiences of women experiencing in vitro fertilisation (IVF) and its impact upon perinatal mental health, drawing upon experiences from midwifery practice. Pseudonyms will be used throughout [1].

5.2   Background

The perinatal period is recognised as a time of significant transition resulting in changes to the women's relationship with her partner, family, friends and wider social network [2]. As part of this transition, the woman may also experience emotional changes [3]. In the Mothers and Babies: Reducing Risk through Audits and Confidential Enquiries (MBRRACE) report [4], it states psychiatric reasons are the fifth biggest cause of maternal death. Historically, women with a known mental illness were discouraged to become pregnant and some even sterilised to prevent it [5]; research now suggests birth rates among women with a history of mental illness are increasing [6]. It is essential midwives have the knowledge and skills to care for these women [6]. Following the findings of the MBRRACE report, there has been a developing interest in maternal mental health, although only minor improvements in rates of death from medical and mental health conditions have been noted [4].

5.3   Anxiety Disorder

Generalised anxiety disorder can present in many ways, and both physical and psychological symptoms can be reported [7]. When physical symptoms of anxiety are reported, (e.g. dizziness, palpitations, abdominal pain, shortness of breath, nausea, headaches), it is important to eliminate alternative conditions prior to making a mental health diagnosis [8]. Psychological symptoms include restlessness, a sense of dread, difficulty concentrating and social withdrawal [7].

The effects of antenatal anxiety on both expectant mother and baby can be profound and has been linked to higher risks of stillbirth, premature birth, low birth weight and major congenital abnormalities [9]. Biaggi et al. [9] disregarded studies that included women with pre-existing or pregnancy-related medical conditions, thus generating results examining the effects of mental health, not other medical factors, on the pregnancy outcome, leading to 97 studies included within their analysis.

Women with anxiety are at a higher risk of depression, sleep disruption, preeclampsia, tocophobia and excessive use of antenatal services [9, 10]. Babies born to those with untreated antenatal anxiety are at higher risks of disrupted emotional regulation and impaired cognitive performance during infancy, behavioural and emotional problems [11–15], inflammatory diseases, gastrointestinal conditions [16] and lower brain volumes in areas associated with learning, memory, social, emotional and auditory language processing [17].

The reasons for these correlated adverse outcomes are unknown; however, some have suggested it is due to decreased blood flow to the foetus and/or the increased levels of cortisol associated with anxiety [9]. Cortisol is released in response to stress; normally, this cannot cross the placenta due to an enzyme which breaks down cortisol to the inactive form cortisone, which is not considered to be harmful [18]. The stress linked with anxiety impairs the function of this enzyme, enabling cortisol to cross the placenta, leading to increased levels of cortisol in the foetus and, consequently, the baby at birth [15].

> Emma, a primiparous woman, had undergone ten unsuccessful cycles of IVF prior to a successful cycle leading to the current pregnancy. At 35 weeks, she was diagnosed with pre-eclampsia and admitted to the antenatal ward. She was well supported by her family and partner and had no previous medical or mental health history of note and no familial history of mental health problems. During her admission, Emma would ask questions repeatedly to the same member of staff and others regarding her observations, blood results and cardiotocograph trace and requested additional tests when not clinically indicated. Midwives working on the ward noted she was very anxious and would require the staff to reassure her continuously.

5.4 Midwifery Role in Caring for Women in the Perinatal Period

Midwives must assess signs of normal or worsening mental health as per the Nursing and Midwifery Council (NMC) [1] code of conduct. Midwives, who are generally regarded positively by women [6, 19], provide continuous care to women through a time which exposes them to a higher risk for mental illness [20, 21]; they play a vital role in the maintenance of optimum health for both expectant mother and baby [1]. Hence, topics such as mental health, risk factors, impact of mental health, both emotionally and physically linked with adverse outcomes, and available resources, in addition to the skills to assess, support and provide pertinent referrals, should be of utmost importance to midwives [22]. Perinatal care for all women can be delivered with a holistic, collaborative and woman-centred approach when midwives are well educated and resilient multidisciplinary working is incorporated into everyday practice [6].

5.5 IVF and Mental Illness

IVF is a form of assisted conception where following ovarian stimulation, eggs are collected, fertilised and replaced in the uterus as an embryo [23]. Infertility has been found to be as severe a disorder as cancer [24], and the emotional toll infertility has remains in 20% of women, even after a successful pregnancy and birth [25].

Several studies have confirmed anxiety levels are increased for those requiring IVF [26–32], with anxiety increase directly correlated to the duration of treatment [33–35] and couples under-report negative effects such as poor mental health [26, 36]. 23.2% of women undergoing IVF treatment experience generalised anxiety disorder; the majority of these have moderate levels of anxiety; however, 12% of these suffer from severe anxiety disorder [37, 38].

Resilience, the ability to maintain emotional stability during challenging times of adversity [39], has been found to be lower in women requiring repeat cycles of IVF, thus leading to an increase in anxiety [40]. However, the opposite was found by Repokari et al. [41] Repokari et al. [41] found couples who have more treatments and have a successful outcome are more resilient than couples who conceive naturally, which has been thought to be due to the overwhelming happiness felt by a couple following a long period of infertility [42]. Tendais and Figueiredo [36] found IVF to increase anxiety levels after birth; it is thought this is due to difficulties adjusting with the transition to parenthood challenging coping abilities, and this is supported by Don and Mickelson [43] and French et al. [26]. 37% of couples requiring IVF experienced maladjustment in the postnatal period, with 10% continuing to experience major mental health issues 11–17 years following IVF treatment [33].

Women have reported their antenatal concerns focused around five themes: miscarriage, baby's health, birth, caring for their baby and finances [44]; those who had IVF had significantly higher levels of anxiety regarding the survival and normality of their babies, injuries to the baby during childbirth and separation from babies after birth [29]. As IVF can be a trigger for poor mental health, and mental illnesses can have adverse outcomes on babies, these fears can be realised more often. Despite this, following successful conception arising from IVF, couples are referred to standard antenatal care [26], with no consideration given in the antenatal guidelines [45] for the additional psychological support they may need [26].

The results of the research suggest ongoing psychological therapies to act as a preventative approach against mental illness would be of benefit to all couples following successful infertility treatment [26, 27, 46]. There is a need for further research to determine whether providing psychological support prevents or lessens adverse mental health for couples experiencing pregnancy as a result of IVF. This would provide more proactive care for women as per the recommendations from the MBRRACE report [4].

5.6 Stigma and Perinatal Mental Health

Less than half of those living with mental health illness seek treatment [47], and stigma is the most significant impediment to seeking mental health care [47, 48]. Mental health is stigmatised at three levels: self, social/public and structural [49]. These levels interact with one another, mutually reinforcing the associated stigma [49]. When people with mental illness believe prejudices and discredited stereotypes regarding those with mental illness, this leads to self-stigma [50].

Self-stigma also correlates with public stigma [51], where the perceived public stigma and threat of discrimination due to mental illness, or knowledge of an experience where mental health treatment has been unsuccessful, feeds into self-stigma [50]. Women perceive a higher level of public stigma [51], which could lead to a higher level of self-stigma. Seeman et al. [52] found structural stigma within developed countries, such as the United Kingdom, where beliefs were mental health was akin to physical illness. However, people had less hope of recovery from a mental illness in developed countries than in developing countries (where people believed mental illness is due to the supernatural or punishment of a person's or ancestor's sins) [52].

Addressing stigma is integral to improving mental health care as it can reduce the number of people seeking treatment and increase mental distress [52, 53]. It has been suggested mild to moderate mental health disorders are seen by and diagnosed by primary care providers rather than mental health providers [47]. Midwives therefore need to be confident and competent with mental health care in order to provide holistic care and in the process reduce stigma associated with poor mental health.

Some midwives deemed Emma was difficult to care for, and this impacted on the care for other women due to demanding time from midwives to answer her repeated questions. However, other midwives successfully identified a potential problem and offered referral promptly, although this was declined by Emma. This potential problem was discussed among midwives, with some deeming Emma 'difficult' rather than considering mental health issues.

Pause for reflection:
- Can you think of women you have cared for who may have been judged as being 'difficult or demanding'?
- Consider the language used when communicating about women and how you might challenge misconceptions.
- Consider your own empathic response—we understand why Emma may have been suffering from generalised anxiety disorder, but what communication skills would the midwife require to enhance empathy and understanding?
- How might you reduce stigma in future when caring for women like Emma?

5.7 Midwifery Training in Mental Health

Midwives recognise they care for women with, or at risk of, mental illness but receive little or no education in mental health [6], therefore are unaware of the resources available and possess scant knowledge of the availability or accessibility of appropriate clinicians [6, 54]. Hence, they class screening for mental health as the least important of all skills, remaining unaware of the symbiotic relationship of mental health on physical health [6].

Whilst the results found during a study by McCauley et al. [6], who issued a questionnaire to midwives practising in Australia, may not be applicable to the United Kingdom, similar findings were noticed by Jarrett [54] and Ross-Davie et al. [55] in research conducted on student midwives and registered midwives in the United Kingdom.

Higgins et al. [22] found poor knowledge to influence midwives leading them to stigmatise women with mental illness perceiving them to be demanding, inconvenient to care for, incapable of effective parenting skills, and at risk of harming babies, others or themselves.

When the perinatal period is the highest-risk time in a woman's life for mental illness [4], it is not acceptable that midwives often feel they lack the knowledge to appropriately care for women suffering mental illness [55, 56]. A lack of knowledge or confidence caring for women with ill mental health has been shown to perpetuate stigma [22], thus leading to a barrier to providing excellent care. This leads to core needs not being met.

Whilst midwives are enthusiastic to further their education by enhancing their knowledge and skills [20, 22, 55, 56], the opportunity is not readily available [6, 54]. It is vital midwives have access to continuous education and training to ameliorate perinatal care [4, 57], and this ought to incorporate scope to explore their own personal attitudes and potentially stigmatising views towards women, for the purpose of reducing negative stereotypes and attitudes [3, 20].

Although antenatal anxiety affects between 13% and 21% of women [58], costing £34,811 per woman, the majority of these costs attributed to the adverse outcomes on the infant [59]; antenatal anxiety is often missed [60]. There were 640,370 births in England and Wales in 2019 [61], so at least 80,000 women are affected by anxiety every year. It is therefore essential health professionals are aware of the importance of screening and treating anxiety during pregnancy. In 2016, Bauer et al. [59] said even in well-funded health systems, less than 50% of those with anxiety are detected, and only 10–15% of those detected have effective treatment.

Low detection rates are attributed to two categories, maternal factors and professional factors [62]. Maternal factors are women not confiding in health professionals regarding their mental health; this could be due to stigma, fear of being a 'bad mother', fear of the baby being taken away and not knowing what is normal [8, 62]. Professional factors are health professionals not asking relevant questions due to lack of training or confidence, time constraints or normalising or dismissing symptoms [62].

5.8　Generalised Anxiety Disorder 2-Item (GAD-2) Screening and Guidance

The National Institute for Health and Care Excellence (NICE) [8] guidelines currently suggest health professionals consider using the Generalised Anxiety Disorder 2-item (GAD-2) screening tool as part of a general discussion of women's mental health and wellbeing at the booking appointment. A mental health assessment should be completed at each visit. The NICE [8] guidelines state to ask questions about depression, but only to consider using the GAD-2. The author feels this is inadequate, and the importance of recognising all mental health problems throughout pregnancy should be embedded within training.

To improve detection rates, health professionals should be proactive, screening for mental health at every encounter a woman has with health professionals [8] and asking open questions and responding to cues (poor eye contact, tears, not sleeping when baby sleeps, reports feeling overwhelmed) [62]. Providing it is not perceived as a box-ticking exercise by women, open questions evoke an array of responses, producing data which can be pertinent to care [63].

5.9   Referral and Multidisciplinary Team Approaches

Midwives need to understand why they are asking about mental health, how to encourage women to disclose and what services are available [6]. Also, educating women why midwives screen for mental health and the importance of and risks associated with ill mental health may encourage women to disclose information [6].

Once anxiety disorder has been detected, a referral to mental health providers should be completed, such as to the perinatal mental health service [8]. It is imperative women are aware of this and a shared decision-making approach is taken [8]. Women-centred approach enables the woman to develop trust and confidence in care providers [6].

Pause for Reflection
- Think of who you may make a referral to in your place of work for women experiencing mental health deterioration.
- Who are the providers in your locality, and do you know how to contact them?
- What does the NMC say about referral outside of our sphere of practice?

5.10   Health Promotion and Mental Health

As pregnant women are receptive to health material that benefits them and their families [64, 65], they are likely to respond well to health promotion from midwives [66]. Health promotion is part of the midwife's role [1], and encouraging healthy behaviours such as adequate sleep, regular physical activity, balanced diet and compliance with perinatal care are all important for general and emotional wellbeing [67].

One of the themes women have when experiencing antenatal anxiety is caring for the baby [44]. Making a postnatal care plan during pregnancy, which addresses infant feeding, social support and mental health, can help prepare women be aware of issues following birth [10, 68]. Midwives are ideally placed to encourage and support women and their families to do this [1].

Treatments for anxiety can include self-help techniques, such as mums and babies activities, antenatal/postnatal exercise classes or support groups [10, 62]. On receipt of a referral, mental healthcare providers can consider medication and are also able to provide psychological therapies, for example, cognitive behavioural therapy, counselling, cognitive analytical therapy or interpersonal therapy [62].

A woman's decision to take medication can be affected by stigma [69]. Stepanuk et al. [69] found when women are less susceptible to social stigma, they make a decision regarding the use of medication that is right for them. This provides a further cause for midwives to encourage a reduction in stigma.

5.11   Medication and Anxiety

Lorenzo et al. [70] state that the medications used for anxiety are the most well researched; women worry medications will impact on the foetus whilst not fully comprehending the impact untreated conditions have [69]. It is of note that medications are unable to be tested during pregnancy due to ethical reasons, and thus professionals are reliant on guidelines, data extrapolated from the general population and retrospective data [60]; however, it has been shown that some adverse effects of medication are not statistically significant [71]. McAllister-Williams et al. [60] noted the risk of neonatal adaption syndromes, such as persistent pulmonary hypertension of the neonate; whilst this is often transient, it should be considered when assessing the need for psychotropic medication during pregnancy. A woman's plans to breastfeed should also be considered when commencing medication; the majority of medications are thought to be safe for use whilst breastfeeding [72, 73]. Additionally, if a woman wants to breastfeed and successfully does, this has been shown to be a protective factor against postnatal depression [74], which women with anxiety are already at higher risk of [9].

- Midwives attempted to discuss Emma's mental health with her and her family; however, she reported she felt it was normal and 'everything will be fine when the baby is here'. Consequently, she declined any support for her mental health. In this case, some midwives acted accordingly, identifying a potential need, although perhaps opportunities were missed to educate Emma of the normal range of mental health and potential risks if abnormally high anxiety levels are left untreated.
- Emma's obstetric condition deteriorated and at 35 weeks gestation required a Caesarean section, and her baby was transferred to the Neonatal Intensive Care Unit.

5.12   Conclusions

Antenatal anxiety has the potential to lead to devastating reverberations socially, emotionally and physically for the woman, and these can have a ripple effect through to her family and close relationships [9, 36, 75]. It is therefore appropriate for healthcare professionals to consider and evaluate the needs of the partner and families, with the potential for addressing those needs through providing support and, if necessary, referral to mental health providers or alternative supportive agencies, such as social services [8]. Partners can act as barriers to women accessing help [76], so informing partners and families of the effects of anxiety and providing additional support may assist in reducing stresses placed on relationships [36, 76].

Research has conclusively shown that midwives have an indispensable and absolute responsibility to identify mental health issues and require better training to support them in this role [4, 6, 55, 57].

A further issue raised is the availability of or the provision of psychotherapeutic support for couples undergoing IVF. IVF has been shown to increase the risk of antenatal anxiety; however, support is not routinely available following the assisted conception [26, 27, 33]. In both providing further education for midwives and routine mental health support throughout the perinatal period for all couples requiring IVF, stigma could be reduced [3, 20, 27]. In doing so, this tackles one of the most critical barriers to mental health seeking actions by women and their families. Providing mental health support during the perinatal period, even with a conservative estimate, could save £3 billion for the health service [58, 59, 61], a substantial economic impact.

References

1. Nursing and Midwifery Council (NMC). The code: professional standards of practice and behaviour for nurses, midwives and nursing associates. London: Nursing and Midwifery Council; 2018.
2. Jonsdottir S, Thorne M, Steingrimsdottir T, Lydsdottir L, Sigurdsson J, Olafsdottir H, Swahnberg K. Partner relationship, social support and perinatal distress among pregnant Icelandic women. Women Birth. 2017;30(1):46–55. https://doi.org/10.1016/j.wombi.2016.08.005.
3. Carroll M, Downes C, Gill A, Monahan M, Nagle U, Madden D, Higgins A. Knowledge, confidence, skills and practices among midwives in the republic of Ireland in relation to perinatal mental health care: the mind mothers study. Midwifery. 2018;64:29–37. https://doi.org/10.1016/j.midw.2018.05.006.
4. Knight M, Bunch K, Tuffnell D, Jayakody H, Shakespeare J, Kotnis R, on behalf of Mothers and Babies: Reducing Risk through Audits and Confidential Enquiries (MBRRACE), et al., editors. Saving lives, improving mothers' care—lessons learned to inform maternity care from the United Kingdom and Ireland confidential enquiries into maternal deaths and morbidity 2014–2016. Oxford: National Perinatal Epidemiology Unit, University of Oxford; 2018.
5. Krumm S, Becker T. Subjective views of motherhood in women with mental illness–a sociological perspective. J Ment Health. 2006;15(4):449–60. https://doi.org/10.1080/09638230600801470.

6. McCauley K, Elsom S, Muir-Cochrane E, Lyneham J. Midwives and assessment of perinatal mental health. J Psychiatr Ment Health Nurs. 2011;18(9):786–95. https://doi.org/10.1111/j.1365-2850.2011.01727.x.
7. National Health Service. Generalised anxiety disorder in adults. [Internet] 2018 [cited 2020 Jul 28]. http://www.nhs.uk/conditions/generalised-anxiety-disorder/
8. National Institute for Health and Care Excellence (NICE). Antenatal and postnatal mental health: clinical management and service guidance (CG192). [Internet] 2018 [cited 2019 Mar 28]. https://www.nice.org.uk/guidance/CG192
9. Biaggi A, Conroy S, Pawlby S, Pariente C. Identifying the women at risk of antenatal anxiety and depression: a systematic review. J Affect Disord. 2016;191:62–77. https://doi.org/10.1016/j.jad.2015.11.014.
10. Thorsness K, Watson C, LaRusso E. Perinatal anxiety: approach to diagnosis and management in the obstetric setting. Am J Obstet Gynecol. 2018;219(4):326–45. https://doi.org/10.1016/j.ajog.2018.05.017.
11. Davis E, Glynn L, Waffarn F, Sandman C. Prenatal maternal stress programs infant stress regulation. J Child Psychol Psychiatry. 2011;52(2):119–29. https://doi.org/10.1111/j.1469-7610.2010.02314.x.
12. Huiping Z, Shuya S, Qian S, Dan Y, Hongli S, Ding D, et al. Involvement of prolactin in newborn infant irritability following maternal perinatal anxiety symptoms. J Affect Disord. 2018;238(1):526–33. https://doi.org/10.1016/j.jad.2018.05.080.
13. Loomans E, van der Stelt O, van Eijsden M, Gemke R, Vrijkotte T, Van den Bergh B. High levels of antenatal maternal anxiety are associated with altered cognitive control in five-year-old children. Dev Psychobiol. 2012;54(4):441–50. https://doi.org/10.1002/dev.20606.
14. O'Connor T, Heron J, Golding J, Glover V, The Avon Longitudinal Study of Parents and Children Study Team. Maternal antenatal anxiety and children's behavioural/emotional problems in children: a test of programming hypothesis. J Child Psychol Psychiatry. 2003;44(7):1025–36. https://doi.org/10.1111/1469-7610.00187.
15. Sandman C, Davis E, Buss C, Glynn L. Exposure to prenatal psychobiological stress exerts programming influences on the mother and her fetus. Neuroendocrinology. 2012;95(1):8–21. https://doi.org/10.1159/000327017.
16. Krause L, Einsle F, Petzoldt J, Wittchen H, Martini J. The role of maternal anxiety and depressive disorders prior to and during pregnancy and perinatal psychopathological symptoms for early infant diseases and drug administration. Early Hum Dev. 2017;109:7–14. https://doi.org/10.1016/j.earlhumdev.2017.03.009.
17. Buss C, Davis E, Muftuler L, Head K, Sandman C. High pregnancy anxiety during mid-gestation is associated with decreased gray matter density in 6-9 year-old children. Psychoneuroendocrinology. 2010;35(1):141–53. https://doi.org/10.1016/j.psyneuen.2009.07.010.
18. Murray I, Hassall J. Change and adaptation in pregnancy. In: Fraser D, Cooper M, editors. Myles textbook for midwives. 15th ed. London: Churchill-Livingstone; 2009. p. 189–225.
19. Feeley N, Bell L, Hayton B, Zelkowitz P, Carrier M. Care for postpartum depression: what do women and their partners prefer? Perspect Psychiatr Care. 2015;52(2):120–30. https://doi.org/10.1111/ppc.12107.
20. Noonan M, Jomeen H, Galvin R, Doody O. Survey of midwives' perinatal mental health knowledge, confidence, attitudes and learning needs. Women Birth. 2018;31(6):358–66. https://doi.org/10.1016/j.wombi.2018.02.002.
21. Wisner K, Austin P, Bowen A, Cantwell R, Glangeaud-Freudenthal C. International approaches to perinatal mental health screening as a public health priority. In: Milgrom J, Gemmill A, editors. Identifying perinatal depression and anxiety evidence-based practice in screening, psychosocial assessment, and management. Oxford: Wiley Blackwell; 2015. p. 193–209.
22. Higgins A, Carroll M, Sharek D. Impact of perinatal mental health education on student midwives' knowledge, skills and attitudes: a pre/post evaluation of a module of study. Nurse Educ Today. 2016;36:364–9. https://doi.org/10.1016/j.nedt.2015.09.007.

23. National Institute for Health and Care Excellence (NICE). Fertility problems: assessment and treatment (CG156). [Internet] 2017. [cited 2020, Jul, 28]. https://www.nice.org.uk/guidance/CG156
24. Cousineau T, Domar A. Psychological impact of infertility. Best Pract Res Clin Obstet Gynaecol. 2007;21(2):293–308. https://doi.org/10.1016/j.bpobgyn.2006.12.003.
25. Poikkeus P, Saisto T, Unkila-Kallio L, Punamaki R, Repokari L, Vilska S, et al. Fear of childbirth and pregnancy-related anxiety in women conceiving with assisted reproduction. Obstet Gynecol. 2006;108(1):70–6. https://doi.org/10.1097/01.AOG.0000222902.37120.2f.
26. French L, Sharp D, Turner K. Antenatal needs of couples following fertility treatment: a qualitative study in primary care. Br J Gen Pract. 2015;65(638):570–7. https://doi.org/10.3399/bjgp15X686473.
27. Garcia-Blanco A, Diago V, Hervás D, Ghosn F, Vento M, Cháfer-Pericás C. Anxiety and depressive symptoms, and stress biomarkers in pregnant women after in vitro fertilization: a prospective cohort study. Hum Reprod. 2018;33(7):1237–46. https://doi.org/10.1093/humrep/dey109.
28. Hashemieh C, Samani L, Taghinejad H. Assessment of anxiety in pregnancy following assisted reproductive technology (ART) and associated infertility factors in women commencing treatment. Iran Red Crescent Med J. 2013;15(12):14465. https://doi.org/10.5812/ircmj.14465.
29. McMahon C, Ungerer J, Beaurepaire J, Tennant C, Saunders D. Anxiety during pregnancy and fetal attachment after in-vitro fertilization conception. Hum Reprod. 1997;12(1):176–82. https://doi.org/10.1093/humrep/12.1.176.
30. Su T, Tzeng Y, Kuo P. The anxiety of Taiwanese women with or without continuity treatment after previous in vitro fertilisation failure. J Clin Nurs. 2011;20(15–16):2217–23. https://doi.org/10.1111/j.1365-2702.2011.03730.x.
31. Ramezanzadeh F, Aghssa M, Abedinia N, Zayeri F, Khanafshar N, Shariat M, Jafarabadi M. A survey of relationship between anxiety, depression and duration of infertility. BMC Womens Health. 2004;4(1):9. https://doi.org/10.1186/1472-6874-4-9.
32. Verhaak C, Smeenk J, Evers A, Kremer J, Kraaimaat F, Braat D. Women's emotional adjustment to in vitro fertilisation: a systematic review of 25 years of research. Hum Reprod Update. 2007;13(1):27–36. https://doi.org/10.1093/humupd/dml040.
33. Gameiro S, van den Belt-Dusebout A, Smeenk J, Braat D, van Leeuwen F, Verhaak C. Women's adjustment trajectories during in vitro fertilisation and impact on mental health 11–17 years later. Hum Reprod. 2016;31(8):1788–98. https://doi.org/10.1093/humrep/dew131.
34. Gourounti K, Anagnostopoulos F, Lykeridou K. Coping strategies as psychological risk factor for antenatal anxiety, worries and depression among Greek women. Arch Womens Ment Health. 2013;16(5):353–61. https://doi.org/10.1007/s00737-013-0338-y.
35. Hassanzadeh M, Khadivzadeh T, Badiee S, Esmaily H, Amirian M. Factors influencing anxiety in infertile women undergoing in vitro fertilisation/intracytoplasmic sperm injection treatment. JMRH. 2018;6(2):1282–8. https://doi.org/10.22038/jmrh.2018.10450.
36. Tendais I, Figueiredo B. Parents' anxiety and depression symptoms after successful infertility treatment and spontaneous conception: does singleton/twin pregnancy matter? Hum Reprod. 2016;31(10):2303–12. https://doi.org/10.1093/humrep/dew212.
37. Chen T, Chang S, Tsai C, Juang K. Prevalence of depressive and anxiety disorders in an assisted reproductive technique clinic. Hum Reprod. 2004;19(10):2313–8. https://doi.org/10.1093/humrep/deh414.
38. Yassini M, Khalili M, Hashemian Z. The level of anxiety and depression among Iranian infertile couples undergoing in vitro fertilization or intra cytoplasmic sperm injection cycles. J Res Med Sci. 2005;10(6):358–62. [Internet]. [cited 2020 Aug 2] https://www.researchgate.net/publication/41390660_The_Level_of_Anxiety_and_Depression_Among_Iranian_Infertile_Couples_Undergoing_In_Vitro_Fertilization_or_Intra_Cytoplasmic_Sperm_Injection_Cycles
39. Rutter M. Implications of resilience concepts for scientific understanding. Ann N Y Acad Sci. 2006;1094(1):1–12. https://doi.org/10.1196/annals.1376.002.

40. Turner K, Reynolds-May M, Zitek E, Tisdale R, Carlisle A, Westphal L. Stress and anxiety scores in first and repeat in vitro fertilisation cycles. A pilot study. PLoS One. 2013;8(5):63743. https://doi.org/10.1371/journal.pone.0063743.
41. Repokari, L., Punamaki, R., Poikkeus, P., Vilska, S., Unkila-Kallio, L., Sinkkonen, J., ..., Tulppala, M. The impact of successful assisted reproduction treatment on female and male mental health during transition to parenthood: a prospective controlled study. Hum Reprod. 2005; 20(11),:3238–3247. https://doi.org/10.1093/humrep/dei214
42. Jongbloed-Pereboom M, Middelburg K, Heineman M, Bos A, Haadsma M, Hadders-Algra M. The impact of in vitro fertilisation/intracytoplasmic sperm injection on parental well-being and anxiety 1 year after childbirth. Hum Reprod. 2012;27(8):2389–95. https://doi.org/10.1093/humrep/des163.
43. Don B, Mickelson K. Relationship satisfaction trajectories across the transition to parenthood among low-risk parents. J Marriage Fam. 2014;76(3):677–92. https://doi.org/10.1111/jomf.12111.
44. Guardino CM & Dunkel Schetter C. Understanding pregnancy anxiety: concepts, correlates and consequences. Zero to Three. 2014 Mar [cited 2020 Aug 2]; 12–21. http://cds.psych.ucla.edu/documents/Guardino_Schetter.pdf
45. National Institute for Health and Care Excellence (NICE). Antenatal care for uncomplicated pregnancies (CG62). [Internet] 2019 [cited 2020 Aug 2]. https://www.nice.org.uk/guidance/CG62
46. Gameiro S, Boivin J, Dancet E, de Klerk C, Emery M, Lewis-Jones C, et al. European Society of Human Reproduction and Embryology guideline: routine psychosocial care in infertility and medically assisted reproduction—a guide for fertility staff. Hum Reprod. 2015;30(11):2476–85. https://doi.org/10.1093/humrep/dev177.
47. Sickel A, Seacat J, Nabors N. Mental health stigma: impact on mental health treatment attitudes and physical health. J Health Psychol. 2016;24(5):586–99. https://doi.org/10.1177/1359105316681430.
48. Corrigan P, Druss B, Perlick D. The impact of mental illness stigma on seeking and participating in mental health care. Psychol Sci Public Interest. 2014;15(2):37–70. https://doi.org/10.1177/1529100614537398.
49. Corrigan P, Kerr A, Knudsen L. The stigma of mental illness: explanatory models and methods for change. Appl Prev Psychol. 2005;11(3):179–90. https://doi.org/10.1016/j.appsy.2005.07.001.
50. Thornicroft G, Mehta N, Clement S, Evans-Lacko S, Doherty M, Rose D, et al. Evidence for effective interventions to reduce mental-health-related stigma and discrimination. Lancet. 2016;387(10023):1123–32. https://doi.org/10.1016/S0140-6736(15)00298-6.
51. Jennings K, Cheung J, Britt T, Goguen K, Jeffirs S, Peasley A, Lee A. How are perceived stigma, self-stigma, and self-reliance related to treatment-seeking? A three-path model. Psychiatr Rehabil J. 2015;38(2):109–16. https://doi.org/10.1037/prj0000138.
52. Seeman N, Tang S, Brown A, Ing A. World survey of mental illness stigma. J Affect Disord. 2016;190(15):115–21. https://doi.org/10.1016/j.jad.2015.10.011.
53. Clement S, Schauman O, Graham T, Maggioni F, Evans-Lacko S, Bezborodovs N, et al. What is the impact of mental health-related stigma on help-seeking? A systematic review of quantitative and qualitative studies. Psychol Med. 2015;45(1):11–27. https://doi.org/10.1017/S0033291714000129.
54. Jarrett P. Student midwives' knowledge of perinatal mental health. Br J Midwifery. 2015;23(1):32–9. https://doi.org/10.12968/bjom.2015.23.1.32.
55. Ross-Davie M, Elliott S, Sarkar A, Green L. A public health role in perinatal mental health: are midwives ready? Br J Midwifery. 2006;14(6):330–4. https://doi.org/10.12968/bjom.2006.14.6.21181.

56. Higgins A, Downes C, Monahan M, Gill A, Lamb S, Carroll M. Barriers to midwives and nurses addressing mental health issues with women during the perinatal period: the mind mothers study. J Clin Nurs. 2018;27(9–10):1872–83. https://doi.org/10.1111/jocn.14252.
57. Coates D, Foureur M. The role and competence of midwives in supporting women with mental health concerns during the perinatal period: a scoping review. Health Soc Care Community. 2019;27(4):e389–405. https://doi.org/10.1111/hsc.12740.
58. Kendig S, Keats J, Hoffman M, Kay L, Miller E, Moore Simas T, et al. Consensus bundle on maternal mental health: perinatal depression and anxiety. J Obstet Gynecol Neonatal Nurs. 2017;46(2):272–81. https://doi.org/10.1016/j.jogn.2017.01.001.
59. Bauer A, Knapp M, Parsonage M. Lifetime costs of perinatal anxiety and depression. J Affect Disord. 2016;192:83–90. https://doi.org/10.1016/j.jad.2015.12.005.
60. McAllister-Williams R, Baldwin D, Cantwell R, Easter A, Gilvarry E, Glover V, et al. British Association for Psychopharmacology consensus guidance on the use of psychotropic medication preconception, in pregnancy and postpartum. J Psychopharmacol. 2017;31(5):519–52. https://doi.org/10.1177/0269881117699361.
61. Office for National Statistics. Statistical bulletin: Births in England and Wales: 2019. [Internet] 2020 [cited 2020 Aug 15]. https://www.ons.gov.uk/peoplepopulationandcommunity/birthsdeathsandmarriages/livebirths/bulletins/birthsummarytablesenglandandwales/2019
62. Shakespeare J. Practical implications for primary care of the National Institute for Health and Care Excellence guideline CG192 Antenatal and postnatal mental health. Royal College of General Practitioners & Maternal Mental Health Alliance. [Internet] 2015 [cited 2020 Aug 15]. http://tvscn.nhs.uk/wp-content/uploads/2015/07/RCGP-Ten-Top-Tips-Nice-Guidance-June-2015.ashx_.pdf
63. Abbott L. The aims of antenatal care. In: Peale I, Hamilton C, editors. Becoming a midwife in the 21st century, vol. 2008. Chichester: John Wiley & Sons Limited; 2008. p. 30–45.
64. Public Health England. All our health: about the framework. London: Public Health England; 2018.
65. United Kingdom Department of Health. Tackling health inequalities: consultation on a plan for delivery. London: Her Majesty's Stationery Office; 2001.
66. Lee D, Haynes C, Garrod D. Exploring the midwife's role in health promotion practice. Br J Midwifery. 2012;20(3):178–86. https://doi.org/10.12968/bjom.2012.20.3.178.
67. Accortt E, Wong M. It is time for routine screening for perinatal mood and anxiety disorders in obstetrics and gynecology settings. Obstet Gynecol Surv. 2017;72(9):553–68. https://doi.org/10.1097/OGX.0000000000000477.
68. Stuebe A, Auguste T, Gulati M. American College of Obstetricians and Gynecologists. Presidential task force on redefining the postpartum visit committee on obstetric practice optimizing postpartum care. Committee Opinion 736. Obstet Gynecol. 2018;131(5):140–50. https://doi.org/10.1097/AOG.0000000000002633.
69. Stepanuk KM, Fisher KM, Wittmann-Price R, Posmontier B, Bhattacharya A. Women's decision-making regarding medication use in pregnancy for anxiety and/or depression. J Adv Nurs. 2013;69(11):2470–80. https://doi.org/10.1111/jan.12122.
70. Lorenzo L, Byers B, Einarson A. Antidepressant use in pregnancy. Expert Opin Drug Saf. 2011;10(6):883–9. https://doi.org/10.1517/14740338.2011.583917.
71. Huber L, Wiley S. Birth outcomes after maternal use of medications for mental health illnesses during pregnancy. Ann Epidemiol. 2007;17(9):749. https://doi.org/10.1016/j.annepidem.2007.07.079.
72. Hale T. Hale's medications and mothers' milk: a manual of lactational pharmacology. 18th ed. New York: Springer Publishing Company; 2019.

73. Jones W. Anxiety and breastfeeding. The Breastfeeding Network: Edinburgh; 2017. https://www.breastfeedingnetwork.org.uk/wp-content/dibm/anxiety%20and%20 breastfeeding.pdf
74. Borra C, Iacovou M, Sevilla A. New evidence on breastfeeding and postpartum depression: the importance of understanding women's intentions. Matern Child Health J. 2014;19(4):897–907. https://doi.org/10.1007/s10995-014-1591-z.
75. Bradley R, Slade P. A review of mental health problems in fathers following the birth of a child. J Reprod Infant Psychol. 2011;29(1):19–42. https://doi.org/10.1080/0264683 8.2010.513047.
76. Fonseca A, Canavarro M. Women's intentions of informal and formal help-seeking for mental health problems during the perinatal period: the role of the perceived encouragement from the partner. Midwifery. 2017;50:78–85. https://doi.org/10.1016/j.midw.2017.04.001.

The Complex Issues of the Perinatal Woman Experiencing Homelessness

Suzanne Reynolds

Abstract

Research surrounding the experiences and impact of women experiencing homelessness during pregnancy is limited, yet the impact of an out-of-home situation on the mother and developing child is far-reaching affecting physical, mental and emotional wellbeing. The legal duty placed on public bodies through the Homelessness Reduction Act to refer people who are at risk of becoming or actually homeless extends to maternity services, yet there is little guidance for midwives on how to support pregnant women experiencing homelessness. Under the umbrella term of homelessness, we will consider not only women residing in hostels or experiencing street homelessness but those living in insecure or inadequate accommodation. Conceptualising homelessness in this way offers a more inclusive approach, highlighting that homelessness is not limited to people living rough and therefore publicly more visible (Amore et al. European Journal of Homelessness. 5:19–37, 2011) but that the impact is far more reaching and detrimental than simply requiring a roof over one's head. This chapter is an exploration of the legal frameworks and social issues that influence the pathway that the pregnant woman may take through homelessness and the effect an out-of-home situation has on the pregnancy, birth outcomes and child development and offers recommendations for good clinical practice within maternity services.

Keywords

Homelessness · Pregnancy · Vulnerable women · Care provision · Temporary accommodation

S. Reynolds (✉)
University Hospitals Birmingham NHS Foundation Trust, c/o Maternity Safeguarding Office, Princess of Wales Maternity Unit, Heartlands Hospital, Birmingham, UK
e-mail: suzannereynolds1@nhs.net

> **Discussion point:** What would you consider as insecure or inadequate accommodation?

Data relating to the numbers of pregnant women who are experiencing homelessness proves problematic to accurately locate. 3820 pregnant women in England [1] and 126 in Wales were accepted for homelessness assistance by local authorities [2] in 2017; however, homelessness datasets in England and Wales use the outcome measure of households where a member is pregnant without dependent children. These figures clearly omit data regarding pregnant women presenting with children and only provide insight into those women who have approached the authorities for help. Many more pregnant women will be hidden from official homelessness statistics through their reliance on family or friends for temporary accommodation prior to seeking assistance [3, 4].

The numbers of women experiencing homelessness, and particularly rough sleeping, are growing [5] prompting increasing discussion and research across varying sectors [6–8], yet there is limited research that explores the impact that homelessness has on pregnant women. It has been suggested that the complex issues of single-person homelessness receive attention due to the high visibility of rough sleepers [9]; therefore, the absence of large numbers of pregnant women on the streets and obscurity within the statistical data may account for the paucity of literature. It is recognised that there is little research surrounding women's needs or experiences whilst sleeping rough, in comparison to that focused upon men [10]. Instead, the studies and reports that do exist appear to concentrate on family homelessness and the impact on parenting behaviour [11–16] or the experiences of children [17–19]. Of the literature that does encompass the impact of homelessness upon pregnancy, there is a predominance of research papers originating from the USA, which may be due to lack of funding into homelessness research within the UK [20]. Subsequently, evidence to form a platform of best practice surrounding care for the homeless perinatal woman has proved challenging to establish.

6.1 Overview of the Legal Framework Surrounding Homelessness and their Implications for Pregnancy

The statutory definition of a homeless person, as set out in Part VII of the Housing Act 1996 [21], is:

1. A person is homeless if he has no accommodation available for his occupation, in the United Kingdom or elsewhere, which he:
   (a) is entitled to occupy by virtue of an interest in it or by virtue of an order of a court,
   (b) has an express or implied licence to occupy, or,

(c) occupies as a residence by virtue of any enactment or rule of law giving him the right to remain in occupation or restricting the right of another person to recover possession.
2. A person is also homeless if he has accommodation but-.
   (a) he cannot secure entry to it, or,
   (b) it consists of a moveable structure, vehicle or vessel designed or adapted for human habitation and there is no place where he is entitled or permitted both to place it and to reside in it.
3. A person shall not be treated as having accommodation unless it is accommodation which it would be reasonable for him to continue to occupy.

It is sometimes, however, easier to conceptualise homelessness as being:
- Roofless: people living rough or in night shelters.
- Houseless: people in hostels, temporary accommodation, refuges, or.
- Living in insecure or inadequate housing: sofa surfing, under the threat of eviction, living under the threat of violence or in severe overcrowding [22].

6.1.1 The Homelessness Reduction Act 2017 and Duty to Refer

The Homelessness Reduction Act [23] came into force in 2017 placing new legal duties on English city councils to strengthen homelessness prevention and to act early in offering support to those threatened with homelessness. The Duty to Refer contained within this Act was developed as part of the wider homelessness reform and is intended to help people get access to homelessness services as soon as possible so their out-of-home situation can be prevented or relieved in a timely manner.

Specified public bodies are required, by law through the Duty, to identify and refer service users to a local authority if they are homeless or threatened with homelessness. The public authorities which are subject to the Duty to Refer are specified in the Homelessness (Review Procedure) Regulations 2018 [24]. Maternity services are considered to be included within the Emergency Departments and Urgent Treatment Centres (e.g. labour wards or maternity assessment centre) or within hospitals as part of their function of providing inpatient care.

There is no requirement when making a referral to have assessed a person's circumstances against the legal meaning of homelessness or threatened homelessness. The opinion of an individual or body making the referral that someone *could* be homeless, or is *possibly* threatened with homelessness, is enough of a reason for it to be made [25]. A referral can only be made with a person's consent, to both the referral itself and the disclosure of their contact details to a local housing authority. The local housing authority is then notified of the reason for the referral and how the individual may be contacted. A 'prevention' duty should be owed to any person who is eligible and threatened with homelessness within the next 56 days.

Where prevention of the homelessness situation is not possible, or the person is already homeless, eligible and has a local connection, the local authority has a duty to provide the person with 56 days in 'relief' duty. Once an applicant has been in relief duty for 56 days, local authorities are required to decide on whether they are owed a main housing duty. Those persons who are eligible, unintentionally homeless, and of priority need are owed the main duty.

- **Discussion point:** What is the process in your Trust for midwives to undertake the Duty to Refer?
- If there is not a documented process, why do you think that might be?

6.1.2 Pregnancy as a Priority Need for Accommodation

Section 193(2) of the 1996 Housing Act requires housing authorities to secure accommodation for applicants who have a priority need. Section 189(1) of the 1996 Housing Act and the Homelessness (Priority Need for Accommodation) (England) Order 2002 [26] states that pregnant women have a priority need for accommodation.

Chapter 8 of the Homelessness code of guidance for local authorities [27] offers a full description of what this means for a pregnant woman:

- 8.5: A pregnant woman, and anyone with whom she lives or might reasonably be expected to live, has a priority need for accommodation. This is regardless of the length of time that the woman has been pregnant. Normal confirmation of pregnancy, e.g. a letter from a medical professional, such as a midwife, should be adequate evidence of pregnancy. If a pregnant woman suffers a miscarriage or terminates her pregnancy before a decision is reached as to whether she is owed section 193(2) main housing duty the housing authority should consider whether she continues to have a priority need as a result of some other factor (e.g. she may be vulnerable as a result of another special reason).

Some hostels and shared accommodation for single persons (without dependants) experiencing homelessness may not be suitable or accept women who are pregnant over a certain gestation. This is commonly around 7 months, and at this time, the housing provider will dispense a Section 8 possession notice [28] (or more commonly known as a *notice to quit*), usually owing to the fact that pregnancy would be in breach of the tenancy agreement. Once a Section 8 notice is provided, the pregnant woman will need to approach her local authority for homelessness assistance.

Authorities have an absolute duty to secure accommodation only for households who are deemed to be unintentionally homeless, and in priority need however, a pregnant woman may have to spend time in temporary accommodation, with the duration and accommodation reliant on the availability of suitable accommodation to the local authority [29]. Unfortunately, being afforded priority need status for housing does not translate directly to speed at which a pregnant woman in an out-of-home situation is allocated housing, nor to the suitability of accommodation that will meet the needs of the pregnant woman or newborn.

The options that may be available can range from hostels, refuges or more supported accommodations to private hotels, B&Bs or other forms of private shared housing [30]. Emergency and temporary accommodation can be located in isolated, unfamiliar or undesirable areas which are not on public transport routes, which can be challenging for women who do not drive, and often have inflexible rules that disallow any visitors to the rooms contributing further to social isolation and loneliness [31]. Different types of homeless accommodation provide different levels of facilities for families, but many lack important equipment and facilities that they need to meet the most basic needs and live healthy lives [18] (Fig. 6.1).

The Homelessness (Suitability of Accommodation) (England) Order 2003 [32] is clear on the use of bed and breakfast accommodation for homeless applicants. The Order specifies it is not suitable for applicants with family commitments (e.g. pregnant women, persons residing with pregnant women, or those with dependent children) due to the lack of cooking and laundry facilities. It is also clearly stated that B&B accommodation should only be used as a last resort to a maximum of 6 weeks' duration. Over the decade, the number of those households that include dependent children or pregnant women has increased with collated figures documenting that 2560 households (including pregnant women) were in B&B style accommodation at the end of June 2018 in England, 900 having resided there for over 6 weeks [33].

There are several instances where the ruling from the Order can be put aside, either there is no alternative housing that the council has available to offer or the Local Authority, housing association or charity owns or manages the accommodation [34]. The former takes into account the current housing crisis and finite resources, whereas the latter suggests that this is the underlying reason why many families can be found in unsuitable temporary accommodation for much longer than is legally allowed. Furthermore, declines in affordable housing, availability of social

---

- Located in unfamiliar, isolated or undesirable areas
- Insufficient or complete lack of cooking facilities
- Shared bathroom facilities with other families with facilities poor or inadequate
- Insufficient or complete lack of laundry facilities
- Lack of available space and privacy - rooms are often small with whole families sharing one room
- Temporary accommodation can be poorly maintained, meaning that families live in housing where there is damp, mould or infestations
- Imposition of rules and lack of flexibility – unable to have visitors leading to social isolation

---

Fig. 6.1 The impact of living in emergency or temporary accommodation

housing, caps to Local Housing Allowance and reluctance of landlords to accept benefits payments [18] consign the most vulnerable to temporary accommodation as housing supplies diminish.

> **Discussion point:** How would you advise and offer support to a pregnant or newly postnatal woman who has been placed in emergency or temporary accommodation?

6.2 Women with no Recourse to Public Funds

No recourse to public funds (NRPF) is a condition imposed on someone due to their immigration status. People with No Recourse to Public Funds imposed conditions are at a higher risk of homelessness or unsafe housing conditions and destitution as they are unable to access local authority housing or welfare benefits [35]. Recent research suggests that around 1.4 million people who are living in the UK are subject to this condition as part of their immigration status, with people from BAME communities most likely to be affected [36]. Section 115 of the Immigration and Asylum Act 1999 [37] states that a person will have 'no recourse to public funds' if they are 'subject to immigration control'. The general policy is that 'those seeking to establish their family life in the UK must do so on a basis that prevents burdens on the taxpayer and promotes integration'. This approach is set out in legislation under Part 5A of the Nationality, Immigration and Asylum Act 2014 [38]. Section 117B(3) states that:

- It is in the public interest, and in particular in the interests of the economic well-being of the United Kingdom, that persons who seek to enter or remain in the United Kingdom are financially independent, because such persons:
  (a) are not a burden on taxpayers, and,
  (b) are better able to integrate into society.

Not having recourse to public funds may not cause an issue, and migrants with this status are able to support themselves through work; however, it is those who are no longer or have never been self-sufficient or whose immigration status has changed or was never regularised where there can be problems. Examples of public funds can be found in Fig. 6.2.

6.2.1 Asylum-Seeking Women

Women who have applied for asylum or are refused asylum seekers are excluded from being able to undertake work or accessing welfare benefits and are unable to approach a local authority for help or an allocation of housing if they are homeless.

Fig. 6.2 Examples of
public funds

Income-based jobseeker's allowance	Income support
Universal credit	Working tax credit
Income-based employment and support allowance (ESA)	
A social fund payment – **includes Sure Start maternity grant**	
Child tax credit	Child benefit
Local authority homelessness assistance	Housing benefit
An allocation of local authority housing	
Council tax benefit	

They are also unable to receive housing benefit to support them in paying rent on a property. Within England, immigration checks also apply to those people who wish to privately rent, and women who are within this category will not have the 'right to rent' and therefore not be accepted as a tenant [39]. However, as an asylum seeker, the woman may be eligible to apply to the Home Office for asylum support, which includes no-choice, basic accommodation if they do not have any other way of supporting themselves [40].

6.2.2 Undocumented Migrant Women

Undocumented migrant women within society are especially vulnerable often being destitute and residing in very precarious situations, with pregnancy compounding their already complex lives and limited survival strategies [41]. Undocumented or 'irregular' migrant women include those who have entered the UK without a visa (e.g. victims of human trafficking or those subject to people smuggling) or have overstayed following the expiry of or made an unsuccessful application of a visa. They may already be dependent upon friends for financial support and accommodation and due to their undocumented status are more likely to become street homeless or sexually abused where favours are exchanged for accommodation [42]. These women should be encouraged to seek specialist immigration advice, or in the case of women who have been victims of trafficking or modern slavery, they should be offered referral into the National Referral Mechanism to obtain support and accommodation through a First Responder organisation [43].

6.2.3 Women on Spouse or Family Visas

Many women who enter the UK on their partner's visa rely on their partners (as primary applicants) for leave to remain in the UK. This coupled with financial dependence (they will usually have a NRPF condition on the visa) puts them in a very vulnerable situation [44] and puts the woman at risk of homelessness and destitution if the relationship breaks down.

The Destitution Domestic Violence (DDV) Concession offers migrant women on family visas with 3 months leave outside of immigration rules to be able to apply for access to limited state benefits and temporary housing whilst she considers applying for indefinite leave to remain (LTR) in the UK [45].

6.2.4 Unmet Eligibility Criteria

Some migrants may be unable to access public funds as they are unable to meet the eligibility criteria. At present, EEA nationals are able to move freely within the EEA; however, in order to claim benefits or access social housing, they must have the right to reside which is based on employment or self-sufficiency. The habitual residence test (which applies to both British citizens who have lived abroad and are returning to the UK and those who have never lived in the UK previously) is designed to stop someone claiming social benefits as soon as they enter the UK. Becoming a habitual resident does not occur immediately upon arrival; even with the intention of settling in that country, the person must have taken up residence and lived in the UK for a period of time [46]. When the habitual residence test is applied to housing applications, it is relevant if the person has arrived or returned to live in the UK during the 2 years prior to making the application [47].

6.2.5 Refugees

Any person who is awarded refugee status within the UK is granted the same rights as a British citizen, being able to access public funds. However, the 28-day period between obtaining the decision and the end of any previous asylum support can subsequently lead to financial hardship, homelessness and a period of destitution as a result of the short time frame to negotiate, apply and receive welfare benefits, particularly in view of the 5-week time frame for the payment of Universal Credit.

6.3   Causes of an out-of-Home Situation in Pregnant Women

Women can become homeless during their pregnancy through the following ways:

– A possession order, expiry or termination of a tenancy agreement.
– Rent or mortgage arrears, debt or financial difficulties.
– Relationship breakdown.
– Asked to leave by family or friends.
– Overcrowded or poor housing conditions.
– Domestic abuse and leaving the home for safety.
– Exiting the criminal justice system.
– No recourse to public funds*.
– Being a victim of human trafficking or modern slavery*.

*These women will be directed through other channels to obtain accommodation support.

The leading cause in the increase of statutory homelessness in England between 2009/2010 and 2016/2017 (of around 30%) has been attributed to the loss of short-hold tenancies within the private rented sector [48]. Furthermore, there is usually a history of adversity that contributes to homelessness among women and creates barriers that may impede recovery [5]. Family breakup, conflict with parents and frequent moves have been cited in contributing to an out-of-home situation prior to pregnancies occurring within young women [49, 50]. Other commonalities include the hidden nature of homelessness, violence and trauma, mental health challenges, substance misuse or addiction and poverty [51].

Becoming pregnant whilst already being homeless has been identified as desta-bilizing [50, 52], and for women who may already be experiencing life adversities, the issue of unsuitable or unstable accommodation adds to the vulnerability of the women and complexity and increased risk to her pregnancy. It is already known that the impact of homelessness on a person's health and wellbeing is wide-ranging—a positive correlation can be observed between the length of time in homelessness and its physical and mental effects [53]. However, the impact of an out-of-home situa-tion on the woman and her unborn during pregnancy is a much less researched topic and requires further exploration.

- **Case Study: Jamelia.** Following divorcing from her husband, Jamelia was made to leave the family home with her four children. They moved fre-quently between the homes of friends but found that they were welcomed less as time went on. Jamelia became pregnant; however, the father of the unborn baby was not the father of her other children and not supportive of the pregnancy which ended the relationship. Jamelia's ex-husband told her that he would support her in the care of their children but not the unborn.
- After around 8 months of sofa surfing, Jamelia was made to leave a friend's home and approached the council for help. The family were placed in one room in a B&B and remained there for around 14 weeks until they were moved to a self-contained flat as a temporary measure.
- Jamelia found her homeless situation and lack of support overwhelming, beginning proceedings at around 34 weeks gestation to place her child in the care of the local authority for adoption.

- **Case Study: Isabella.** Isabella was living with her boyfriend; however, when she discovered she was pregnant, he left her, so she moved back to her father's home to be closer to her family: 'So I wanted to come and be closer to family, and it didn't kind of work out exactly to how I planned things. So it was just a bit of a shock to the system… from my dad's - when he kicked me out…'.

- Following an argument when Isabella was 4 months pregnant, Isabella's father made her leave, and so she moved into her uncle's home. This resulted in Isabella sleeping on the sofa as her uncle resided in a one-bed bungalow. Isabella found this difficult as her uncle was also a heavy drinker.
- Isabella was unable to find work and consequently was unable to privately rent. She found it difficult to negotiate with the system, unable to find many resources to support homeless pregnant women, and finally approached the council for help when she was around 30 weeks pregnant.
- Isabella was placed in a local bed and breakfast accommodation, but struggled with being isolated and vulnerable, combined with pre-existing anxiety issues, so she left and returned to her uncle's property when she was 34 weeks pregnant, preferring to be closer to family despite the conditions in the home.
- Isabella felt the whole experience impacted negatively on her pregnancy: *'I was constantly thinking I need to do this and I need to do that, and I need to fix this and I need to make this much, or do this, or just constantly trying to better myself. But just not actually being present in my pregnancy...'.*

- **Case study: Kayla.** Kayla was initially living with her nan. When she found out she was pregnant, she moved in with her partner who still resided with his mother. This arrangement only lasted a month, and the couple were told they needed to leave so they approached the local authority for help when Kayla was around 5 months pregnant.
- They were initially placed out of the local authority area in a Travelodge for two weeks, then were moved back into the area to a hotel used by the council for emergency homelessness accommodation. Kayla commented: *"we went to the room and the door was...it didn't look safe to me, and the door looked like it had been booted down a few times. We only had two kitchens for three floors over and over a hundred rooms on each floor, so we could never ever get into use the kitchen."*
- Kayla contacted the local council because of the conditions: *"I broke down on the phone, and told them that I didn't feel safe there, I didn't want the babby there, I didn't want her there when she was born. Like I didn't want any of us there, and it wasn't safe for me, and there was countless arguing outside our door, there was banging, there was shouting, there was nights where didn't sleep, because of it all."*
- *"Well, they were giving us false hope, basically, because they were saying we'll definitely get you somewhere, you'll definitely be safe, you're definitely a priority..."*
- Kayla remained in the hotel until her daughter was four months old. At this point, the family were offered accommodation through a friend which they accepted.

6.4   Impact on Women's Experiences of Being Homeless and Pregnant

There is a growing body of evidence that supports the deleterious consequences of homelessness on families and the children, yet there is a dearth of literature describing the journey of a pregnant woman into homelessness or specifically the experiences of a homeless pregnant woman. Themes such as instability, stress and lack of control are common [11, 54] with women commenting on the high levels of distress, mental health issues, isolation and lack of social support they experience upon becoming homeless [55]. The author's own research highlighted the mental impact that women felt entering homelessness during pregnancy – initial shock and uncertainty followed by ongoing stress. They also recounted feelings of imprisonment within their rooms due to the location and inflexible rules of the emergency accommodation, leading to their social isolation when they were feeling most vulnerable. Women have also cited a lack of solicitude towards them from frontline workers, inadequate and poorly located accommodation and an absence of dedicated services as challenging their perceptions of pregnancy being a 'priority need' and led women to push aside their pregnancy and not be 'present' to focus on their developing baby [56].

- *'We tried explaining... How were we meant to be a priority if you won't do anything? And they're like, well, you are a priority, but - and I'm like there's no buts, we're either a priority and you're going to help us, or we're not. And, as far as I can tell, they never ever wanted to help, so we obviously wasn't. I mean, I'm not sure how a new born baby isn't a priority, because why do you want to keep them in somewhere like that...?*
- *'I mean, because they don't know you, they don't know your baby... you to think to yourself, okay, well, I don't need to know my baby at the minute, when, in reality you do. And that's how they make you feel, they're like, the baby can wait, it's not like the baby is here... so then you... start thinking, okay, well, maybe they're right and, in reality, they're not, you shouldn't have to feel that way, you shouldn't have to feel you're pushing your pregnancy aside for them...'*—**Case study: Kayla**

Not surprisingly, an out-of-home situation has been found by mothers to have negatively impacted upon their experience of pregnancy on what women believe should be a happy time [11, 54].

'...sometimes I even forget that I was pregnant. You have a little problem, yeah? And when you see more than that problem, you forget the little one, yeah? Sometimes I forget that I was pregnant, even I cannot sit because I was all the day going there, or going to there, there, there...'—**Case study: Rahma**

6.4.1 Impact on Pregnancy and Birth Outcomes

Food insecurity during the period of homelessness is highly prevalent [57]. Multiple moves between accommodations whilst homeless have been demonstrated to require a great deal of personal investment and energy and impacts greatly on their usual food access process [58]. Lack of kitchen facilities, refrigeration or food storage space in temporary accommodation means that pregnant women will often obtain food right before consumption [31, 59], leading to the reliance upon fast foods [56]. Poor nutritional status during pregnancy can negatively influence the timing of birth and birth weight of the foetus [60]. The chronic stress associated with homelessness experienced by pregnant women has also been linked to having a significant impact on preterm birth [61].

- **Discussion point:** Information provided to women during pregnancy should be feasible within the context of their situation.
- Given the barriers identified in maintaining an appropriate diet whilst in emergency or temporary accommodation, how would you discuss maintaining a healthy pregnancy in a situationally specific and culturally sensitive way?

Studies particularly concerned with the impact of homelessness on pregnancy outcomes have demonstrated low birth weight and preterm birth even when controlled for demographic and perinatal variables [62–65] to establish that homelessness during pregnancy is an independent risk factor for adverse birth outcomes. An analysis of birth outcomes using data gathered from women who were homeless during their pregnancy established an association between the out-of-home situation, lower birth weight and a threefold risk in preterm birth [66]. A further large-scale study using maternal health surveillance program data demonstrated a higher prevalence of low birth weight (<2500 g) in babies born to women who were homeless 12 months prior to the birth [67]. Out-of-home situations and housing instability in pregnancy thus appear to contribute significantly to lower birth weight and increase the risk of preterm labour.

6.4.2 Impact on Child Development

There is considerable body of research which demonstrates the damaging effects of homelessness and child development following the birth of the child. The physical loss that is felt by becoming homeless is further compounded by feelings of stress, anxiety, isolation, loss of control, diminishing self-efficacy and potentially self-worth; parents trying to cope with their own histories of adversity can challenge the ability to provide consistent care in a nurturing way to their baby [68]. This has been observed through a decreased ability to sensitively parent [11–14, 17, 69] and a high occurrence of emotional and behavioural problems associated with childhood homelessness [16,

70] to such an extent that homelessness is now being recognised as a significant contributor associated with Adverse Childhood Experiences (ACEs) [71].

Poor and unsuitable housing has been noted to feature regularly in Serious Case Reviews in cases of abuse and neglect [65, 72–74] as homelessness is not routinely considered a safeguarding issue often sitting outside of multi-agency support that the family is receiving [75]; however, this still leaves children vulnerable and susceptible to risk. Further exploration and discussion of the impact on child development is, however, outside of the remit of this chapter.

6.5 Role of the Midwife and Maternity Service Recommendations

An in-depth exploration into the role of the midwife in public health identified that homelessness is a subject that midwives do not tend to discuss with women [76]. Women have previously voiced a perceived stigmatisation due to their homelessness situation [52, 59, 77, 78] which may make them less likely to divulge this information. If the living conditions of the woman who is threatened by or experiencing an out-of-home situation are not divulged or questioned by professionals, a form of collusion occurs and is promoted through non-action—the woman unknowingly becoming a participant in her own neglect [59]. Consequentially, it is important that the signs of homelessness, or those women at risk, can be recognised and referred to the appropriate organisations so that her health and housing needs can be adequately addressed.

There are currently no national UK recommendations or care pathways that specifically focus on the care of a pregnant woman experiencing homelessness. Whilst there is mention of vulnerable women such as those who are homeless, there is no suggestion as to how services may look or be delivered [79, 80]. The Royal College of Midwives [81] suggests that open questions that specifically are related to the woman's current housing situation should be asked on at least four occasions, at booking, at 28 weeks, at 36 weeks and on postnatal discharge, and offers examples of ways to ask these questions in Fig. 6.3. However, if a housing concern is raised at any point in the pregnancy, it should be acted upon. Asking women about their housing situation at their initial booking with maternity services may be the first disclosure they make to professionals that they are homeless. Many women may not be aware of who to approach for help or their rights in this situation; some women may not be homeless at that point, but the circumstances in which they are living may put them at risk.

- **Discussion point:** Consider your particular area of work, how likely are you to provide maternity care for a woman who is or is threatened with homelessness?
- How might you introduce or discuss the topic of secure housing and homelessness with a woman?
- How comfortable would you feel in doing this and offering advice or support?

- How secure is your long-term accommodation?
- Where do you plan to spend the first few weeks with your baby?
- Have you thought about where your baby will sleep?

Fig. 6.3 Ways to open conversations about housing circumstances

- Basic information – name, gender, contact details, address, ethnicity, nationality
- Details of agencies that the person engages with
- The date the person will become homeless
- Details of the person's homelessness situation or threat of homelessness
- Details of the person's other household members
- The person's wishes in the context of the referral
- Any support needs identified
- Any risks that the person could pose
- The pregnancy details or dependent children
- Details of a known physical disability or mental health concerns

Fig. 6.4 Information required by midwives to complete a Duty to Refer on a client

If a pregnant woman discloses that she is, or threatened with homelessness whilst a hospital inpatient, as discussed earlier in this chapter, midwives have a Duty to Refer her to the Local Housing Authority (LHA) for housing advice and assistance if she consents to it. Each local authority will have their own procedure for referral, many using the ALERT housing jigsaw portal. Hospital services may have their own guidance or services, such as a Complex Discharge Team, Homeless Health Practitioner or specialist midwife or nurse within a Safeguarding Team who can help midwives undertake a referral. The information that is required for the referral is included in Fig. 6.4.

6.5.1 Ensuring Engagement with Maternity Services in an out-of-Home Situation

An out-of-home situation can introduce numerous issues that make it more difficult for pregnant women to continue to engage with maternity services (Fig. 6.5). Models of

- Having to move between universal services as they change area, so relationships with professionals i.e.midwives and GPs can break down.

- Women can decide that it is not worth registering temporarily with a GP as they are moved regularly

- Women may struggle to prove eligibility for services and claim benefits due to lack of stable address.

- It can be harder for home visits to take place in temporary accommodation to assess the woman's living situation, especially when she has moved out of the area

- In a new area, families may not know where the services are or how to access them.

- Practical and emotional issues can make it harder for families to engage with services. These include a lack of money to pay for transport, fear of stigma, low confidence and anxiety issues.

- Physical and emotional fatigue experienced due to trying to sort out accommodation, pack up and move on, constantly going out for food, long travelling times.

Fig. 6.5 Issues which make it harder for pregnant women to engage with services

maternity care for women who have health and social inequalities that promote safety as well as personalised care have been recommended in recent reports and government policy [82, 83]. Continuity of care models demonstrate that women who receive midwifery-led continuity of care have improved birth and neonatal outcomes as well as increased satisfaction [84] through midwives being able to take a holistic approach in the woman's care, responding not only to physical needs but to her emotional and social needs [85].

Becoming homeless diverts the woman's priorities away from her pregnancy. Barriers to attending antenatal appointments exist such as transport issues (lack of transport or finances to travel), the location of appointments, unsuitable appointment times (especially either early or later in the day when travelling long distances and having to pick other children up from school) or waiting times [77, 86].

The location of emergency and temporary accommodation can pose additional difficulties to maternity services as they may be situated outside of Trust boundaries where the women is booked for her care. Trusts may also have differing opinions or guidelines regarding home visits. In the author's experience, out-of-area community midwives have refused to carry out an antenatal visit at the woman's temporary accommodation based purely on her difficulty in reaching her named midwife for an antenatal check-up. This disruption in antenatal and/or postnatal care provision may in extreme circumstances threaten the woman's right to safe and appropriate care under Article 2 (right to life) of the Human Rights Act 1989 [87] if she is unable to access specialist services due to the location of the accommodation. Local and public authorities should take this into consideration when making decisions that may ultimately put someone's life in danger [88].

> *'And they put me through far away and I don't know, I'm really stressed, I can't come… Sometimes I have to tell them [midwives] I can't come and I have to ignore the calls. You can't come because you're far away, or you can't come because you're really tired and stressed and you can't go. Or…sometimes you can't go because of the weather and it's cold, you can't…you don't want to go, you're tired of going out, because of the food.'*—**Case study: Ayesha**

In view of the potential impact on the growth of the unborn baby and the increased risk of preterm labour in women who are, or are threatened with homelessness, midwives should make every effort to work with the mother to closely monitor the wellbeing of the unborn baby. Midwives should also consider the mental impact and stress that the situation will have on the mother and routinely ask her about her mental health so that she can be signposted or referred to the relevant support agencies.

If the woman has been moved to a different area due to being housed in emergency or temporary accommodation, discuss temporary registration at a GP surgery that is local to her to assist her in maintaining regular antenatal care and to reduce the likelihood of non-attendance at appointments due to transport or financial issues. If the woman wishes to remain at the same GP surgery, endeavour to arrange antenatal appointments at times that are more suitable to her if she is having to travel long distances. Women can also be provided with a HC5(T) travel refund form to claim travel expenses for hospital appointments.

Establishing good working relationships with community midwifery teams in the areas that are known to be used by the local authority for emergency and temporary accommodation assists in arranging antenatal care at the woman's accommodation and facilitates more effective handover of care.

> **Discussion point:** Consider how maternity care is provided to women within your Trust. Does this support or obstruct engagement with homeless pregnant women?

6.5.2   Support during Pregnancy

If a pregnant woman has been moved into an unfamiliar area or the accommodation she has been placed in has inflexible rules around visitors, a network of professional support can be invaluable to assist in reducing her social isolation and increasing protective factors within the family by alleviating some of the instability and stress [11, 12, 14]. The homeless pregnant women and her family will require increased support from both universal and targeted services owing to the increased vulnerability and additional challenges they are faced with during this time [68].

The actions taken to reduce health inequalities should start before birth, with pregnancy presenting an ideal opportunity for midwives and other allied health professionals to influence the women's lifestyle and maximise life chances [79, 89]. The mental and physical health of a pregnant woman, including her behaviours, relationships and the environment, can have an effect on the intrauterine environment and development of the foetus, thus impacting upon its wellbeing and long-term outcomes (as previously discussed).

Early intervention programmes such as Early Help work to reduce these risks factors and increase the protective factors in a child's life [90]. Parents have a greater chance of being able to offer sensitive and responsive care to their newborn and other children if they have experienced secure attachment relationships themselves, combined with knowledge around child development, supportive relationships and emotional wellbeing [68]. Undertaking an Early Help Assessment with a pregnant woman, where there are concerns around inadequate housing or homelessness, can assist the family to obtain coordinated support from more than one agency (e.g. health, housing, education, police, voluntary support agencies).

Understanding what services are available to women experiencing homelessness in the local and adjacent areas will equip midwives to be able to pull together the appropriate agencies to offer a package of support. This may range from the allocation of a family support worker from a local children's centre or local charities to referral into specialist services offering advice or floating support for homeless families. Housing services are often described as being separate and difficult to access or influence, appearing unresponsive to letters from professionals advocating for their women's needs, and rarely included in multi-agency support [75]. In an area where there are notable numbers of pregnant women experiencing homelessness, striving to develop links with the local authority housing department, in particular those whose main role is to the allocation and movement within temporary accommodation, is invaluable for escalation of issues including length of time spent in a B&B or hotel or trying to arrange a move on into self-contained accommodation prior to the birth.

- **Discussion point:** What services are available local to your Trust that can support pregnant women and families who are homeless?
- Do you know how to refer into them?

Where families are more transient due to their homeless situation, an Early Help approach can be more difficult as professionals involved may change regularly because of the geographical location of the family. However, the provision of *any* social support, parenting support programmes, early identification of mental health issues or support to reduce social isolation can help mitigate some of the negative effects of homelessness whilst attempts are made to resolve the situation. Concern from midwives about the woman's homeless situation can make her feel that someone is there for her.

> *'it was nice to think that someone actually did care…. she understood, and if I wanted to talk to her I could.'*—**Case study: Heidi**

It is not only the programme of support that is offered to women experiencing homelessness that is important but the approach that is taken to deliver it. A trauma-informed approach to care has been advocated as best practice in homeless service settings [91]. An out-of-home situation can be viewed as a traumatic experience, and as previously discussed, many women's lives are intertwined with consequences of previous trauma [92]. Viewing women experiencing homelessness through a 'trauma lens' can help midwives and other professionals involved better understand their behaviours, responses and how they relate to others [93]. Lacking this awareness may increase the risk of additional trauma and harm to the woman. The benefit of adopting an Early Help approach to support trauma-informed practice is that it can help the woman experiencing homelessness regain a sense of self control, as she identifies and drives her own goal setting and can be kept informed of her situation, which are key tenets of trauma-informed care [94].

6.6 The Role of Social Services and the Pregnant Woman Experiencing Homelessness

In the first instance when a pregnant woman enters an out-of-home situation, she should approach the local authority for housing assistance for an assessment and to see if she is owed a duty to be housed. Homelessness is often not regarded as a safeguarding matter, and assessments under the Care Act 2014 or pre-birth assessments under Section 17 of the Children Act 1989 are commonly not undertaken, waiting until the baby is born to decide whether to offer support. Action such as this has been criticized in a serious case review, although it was acknowledged that the complexities surrounding the woman's circumstances and legal frameworks pose a challenge to housing and social care workers across the country [74].

Adult social services may have a role to play if the woman is identified as a potential victim of modern slavery or trafficking. The local authority, as a first responder organisation, must notify the National Referral Mechanism, and should the woman have no recourse to public funds, housing may be available through the NRM. The local authority will also need to consider if they should provide accommodation to prevent a breach of human rights or to comply with the EU Anti-Trafficking Directive under the Localism Act 2011 [95, 96]. However, there should also be consideration of whether accommodation can be provided to the homeless pregnant woman through adult social services under the Care Act 2014, if action is required to prevent or stop abuse and if she has a need for care and support and is unable to protect herself from abuse or neglect due to her needs [97].

Children's social services may have a duty to accommodate children within the family if the pregnant woman is unable to secure accommodation through a homeless application, for example, due to her immigration status or if intentional homelessness has occurred. Section 17 of the Children Act 1989 [98] places a duty on local authorities to provide destitute families with housing and subsistence payments if they are needed to safeguard the welfare of a child in need even if the family does not have recourse to public funds. Therefore, pregnant women with children who are identified to be threatened with or become homeless and are subject to a no recourse to public funds clause should be referred to Children's Services.

There are some exceptions to this: EEA nationals, most refused asylum seekers and undocumented migrants are not entitled to apply for Section 17 support, and where this is the case the local authority has a duty to report these ineligible families to the Home Office [99].

The failure to provide accommodation under the Housing Act 1996 [100] may also prove to be a breach of human rights. This is not due to the actual act of not offering accommodation but the resultant consequences of doing so, for which the local authority must take some degree of accountability for. For example, should the pregnant woman or her family experience or suffer from inhuman or degrading treatment (Article 3: Freedom from torture and inhuman or degrading treatment) [101] that would compromise their right to physical or psychological integrity (Article 8: Respect for your private and family life) through not being offered accommodation, particularly where there is a family unit involved, this could constitute a breach of human rights [102]. Article 8 rights may also be employed if accommodation provided by the local authority is not suitable to the degree that it interferes with a private or family life (e.g. accommodation that is not suitably adapted for a person with disabilities) [103].

- **Case Study: Tambara.** Tambara attended the local maternity unit, pregnant with her first baby at 42 weeks gestation. Although she had been in the UK for over a year, it was her first experience of maternity services and had not booked with any maternity unit until she was around 28 weeks pregnant. She had recently moved from a different county as she had split up with her husband (who was not the father of the unborn baby) and was staying with a friend.
- Following the birth, Tambara informed staff that she was worried about her housing situation, as her friend was living in a one-bedroom flat, which wasn't actually hers, and she had told Tambara she couldn't stay. Tambara did not have any other friends or social support with whom she could stay with.

- Midwifery staff contacted the unit she was previously booked at, and it was discovered that Tambara's visa in the UK had expired, leaving her in a situation unable to approach the local council for help and support. Discussion with Tambara around her immigration circumstances revealed she had applied for leave to remain several months before but had not yet had her claim dealt with and owing to her pregnancy had not been able to work.
- Midwifery staff submitted a Children's Social Services referral to be assessed by the No Recourse to Public Funds team, stating that Tambara is unable to access local authority housing assistance and had the potential to become street homeless with a newborn baby. The impact of Tambara's destitution on the health, wellbeing and provision of clothing and equipment for the newborn baby was documented in the referral, thus invoking Section 17 of the Children Act 1989 and, if this was not adhered to, the breach of their human rights.
- Children's Social Services accepted the case and arranged for Tambara and her newborn baby to be discharged to a hotel commonly used in supporting destitute families after 7 days in the hospital.

6.7   Homelessness at the Time of Birth and within the Postnatal Period

Pregnancy and housing services timelines are becoming increasingly mismatched due to the rising demand for social housing and priorities within the housing system that do not consider the needs of pregnant women experiencing homelessness. Many women may still find themselves in an out-of-home situation at the time of birth, and this lack of resolution renders their priority need status into an empty promise [56].

'I've seen the ladies that… had a baby in there…and they're like 'we've been here for half a year, and I had my baby'. And I literally thought I'm going to have the baby in there. I mean, if she had it I'll be the same, I'll be having the baby in there, so what am I going to do?'—**Case Study: Ayesha**

An exploration of women's birth experiences in London described women who had been discharged from the maternity unit in early labour yet had nowhere safe to return to, labouring elsewhere in the hospital or on the street or discharging women first thing in the morning with a newborn baby in order for them to attend the housing office [75]. These actions call into question whether all reasonable steps had been taken to protect the mothers and babies (who could be seen as vulnerable or at risk from harm, neglect or abuse by not having any accommodation to return to) before discharging them, or if they had taken into consideration respecting and/or upholding their human rights. These are both difficult ethical and clinical judgements to make, with midwives concern for the safety of their patients often being overruled by the need for beds on the wards [104]; however, to not take these issues into account could be seen as directly contravening The Code [105] for standards of care. However, the alternative is that new mothers without any accommodation remain lodged on the postnatal ward for an indefinite period of time, whilst midwives and managers struggle to liaise with housing and/or social services to try to resolve their homelessness situation, thus further highlighting the severity of the housing crisis, lack of rapid referral processes and non-existence of joint working between maternity and local authority housing services.

There do not appear to be any official guidelines, policies or pathways that can advise or assist midwives when faced with the predicaments above. Ideally, if the woman has disclosed the instability of her housing situation to her midwife or other caregiver prior to the birth of the baby, a housing needs assessment will have been instigated through the Duty to Refer and accommodation provided to the woman. However, the Duty to Refer does not prompt an emergency response from the local authority, and although it should be completed, other options will need to be explored for accommodation to be found. The approach (outlined in Fig. 6.6) that the author tentatively puts forward is one that has been discussed at length between the author, her maternity safeguarding matron and two local housing authorities to try to support the midwives' practice and promote a safe discharge of the mother and her newborn baby back into the community.

In cases where the baby is cared for on the Neonatal Unit, the National Maternity Review [83] advocates that parents should be actively encouraged to participate in their baby's care with neonatal services including accommodation and assistance for parents. In units which do provide accommodation, this may prove an invaluable support for mothers who have not been able to resolve any homelessness issues prior to the birth of the baby and offers a safe place to stay whilst she addresses her situation with the local housing authority.

When emergency accommodation is offered in the postnatal period, it will be on a no-choice basis and should be accepted. This does mean that women can be discharged to a bed and breakfast or hotel-type accommodation due to the lack of social housing. There should be liaison between midwifery staff, the local authority and the accommodation provider to ensure that any room in a hotel-type accommodation is on a lower floor and a cot can be provided to encourage safe sleeping practices. It may not always be possible to carry out an inspection of the environment prior to the woman's discharge; therefore, any following visits should aim to address or escalate any concerns found with the accommodation provided. Many hotel- or bed and breakfast-type accommodations do not allow the use of electrical equipment within the rooms, which may add further stress and negatively impact on the chosen feeding method. Where it is known that a woman will be discharged post-natally with her baby to this type of accommodation, it would be prudent to discuss the use of cold water sterilisers so that the mother is not breaching any accommodation agreements.

- If the woman is in early labour, ask about her home circumstances and if she has the means to travel to and from the unit. If there are concerns raised by the woman or midwifery staff, then admission to the unit would be preferable whilst labour establishes.
- Complete the Duty to Refer at point when concerns around homelessness occur, keeping in mind it is not an emergency response.
- If the woman presents with her partner, then the partner should be advised to attend the local housing authority as soon as possible to make a homelessness application and emergency accommodation be arranged.
- If the woman attends on her own, she should be encouraged to telephone the local housing authority to discuss her situation (at the earliest, most convenient time).
- If the woman is unable to do this, maternity staff should contact the local housing authority to begin the process for her.
- Midwifery staff should try to explore all housing options with the woman, to see if there are any friends or family that she could safely stay with in the interim period whilst her accommodation needs are being addressed.
- Midwifery staff should also explore any safeguarding issues that may instigate a referral into Adult or Children's Social Services (for example, if the local housing authority is not an option in the case of women with NRPF, or a homelessness application has been rejected).
- Midwifery staff should bear in mind any breaches to the Code or the woman's human rights when planning her discharge from hospital, using these to support any referrals that are made.
- In extreme circumstances, the woman may be advised to attend the local housing authority herself to be offered emergency accommodation, however this should only be after liaison with the local housing authority and where there is no other option to undertake a homelessness assessment. In this case, a taxi should be provided through the Trust and where possible, the baby accommodated on the ward during this time.
- If the baby is on the neonatal unit, it should be explored with the management if there are any facilities that she could stay in whilst addressing her housing needs and being able to actively participate in her baby's care.

Fig. 6.6 Approach to safe discharge if a homeless situation is disclosed at the time of giving birth or in the immediate postnatal period in hospital

Emergency accommodation, as previously discussed, regularly has inflexible rules regarding visiting; therefore, any support from family or friends will be severely restricted, leaving the new mother on her own in less than satisfactory accommodation. Maternity staff should also ensure that the new mother feels confident in her chosen feeding method and baby cares, and has been observed and supported over several days with these skills if required.

If the mother is entering emergency accommodation from hospital, a discharge planning meeting involving the mother, community midwife, health visitor, housing and any other support service that has been involved with the woman during her pregnancy should be held to ensure that there is clear communication regarding the woman's needs and provides the opportunity for a full handover of care if new professionals will be involved. If professionals are unable to attend in person, this can be carried out virtually or via a telephone conference.

- **Discussion point:** consider how feasible this approach would be within your place of work.
- Are there any improvements you could make? What are the sticking points?

6.8 The Role of a Specialist Midwife for Women Experiencing Homelessness during their Pregnancy

The Better Births document draws attention to the role of health professionals with specialist expertise in improving outcomes for those who are particularly vulnerable, for example, homeless people, asserting that in caring for women, this translates as being able to take the time to listen, determine individual needs and establish whether other referrals are required [83]. Women who have access to specialist midwives have described the positive difference their support has made to their needs [106]. Specialist midwives have the advantage of being able to spend extra time with mothers, developing relationships of trust to be able to address complex needs more fully or recognise confusion and fears to be able to guide women through unfamiliar systems or procedures [107] or to refer to other external agencies for support.

Housing and homelessness legislation is complex, and the skill set and confidence to understand and discuss these issues that has to be developed by a specialist midwife for women experiencing homelessness is, in the author's experience, forged through tenacity, not being afraid to ask questions and continued efforts to establish professional relationships with local authority housing departments and voluntary support agencies.

The recent standards of proficiency for midwives assert the midwife's role in assessment and management of complications and additional care needs, such as homelessness [108]. The appointment of a midwife to this specialist role enables in-house training to be provided to maternity staff and to students to better understand the complex needs of a pregnant woman experiencing homelessness and to develop guidelines to support the care of these women as they enter and move through maternity services, assisting in the achievement of these standards. Time can also be taken to offer support to midwives through discussion of cases, being involved in or leading on Early Help programmes, completing social care referrals and understanding and advocating for the woman's human rights where complexities exist that bar normal pathways from being accessed. Fig. 6.7 offers recommendations for healthcare professionals involved in supporting a pregnant woman experiencing homelessness.

The specialist midwife can also dedicate the time and effort to establish good working relationships with local authority housing departments for the escalation of

- Undergo training on the impact of homelessness in pregnancy on women, the developing fetus and its effect on sensitive parenting
- Have a basic understanding of the Homelessness Reduction Act 2017 and appropriate referral pathways into local authority homelessness services to signpost women who inform them of an unstable or unsuitable housing environment prior to being made homeless
- Understand and be able to provide information to homeless pregnant women about how they can be reimbursed for hospital visits when they are on a low income
- Where there are high rates of homelessness, consider the appointment of a Specialist Midwife for homeless pregnant women to oversee their care and offer specialist signposting and advice

Fig. 6.7 Recommendations for healthcare professionals involved in the care of the pregnant woman experiencing homelessness

concerns surrounding women's circumstances or to understand a woman's situation in more detail. In the author's role, this has been developed into an understanding that she will inform the local authority temporary accommodation department about any pregnant woman who has been in a B&B–/hotel-type accommodation for longer than 6 weeks (or sooner if medical issues such as diabetes have not been taken into account for the placement) or if the woman's gestation is greater than 30 weeks to facilitate move-on into self-contained accommodation prior to the birth.

6.9 Summary

This chapter has attempted to explore the complex issues that impact upon a pregnant woman when she enters a homelessness situation, through discussion of homelessness legislation, limited available research, the role of social services and consideration of human rights. The case studies within the chapter demonstrate women's experiences of homelessness, with points for discussion for the reader to consider what practices and services currently exist or may be required to support pregnant women in an out-of-home situation within their Trust.

It is hoped that the information contained within this chapter can be used to develop local guidelines or pathways within maternity units in order for women experiencing homelessness to be offered equitable care provision. The suggested approach to a care pathway and support, in the absence of national guidelines or recommendations, has been based on the literature available alongside the author's personal experience of providing midwifery care to the pregnant woman experiencing homelessness over the last four and a half as a specialist midwife and undertaking research in this area.

One thing is clear, the implications of women entering homelessness during their pregnancy are far-reaching and long-lasting, not only for the woman but to the health and development of the child. Midwives and allied healthcare professionals have a key role in identifying pregnant women who are threatened with, or are actually homeless, enabling them to access local authority assistance and helping to provide a package of support to mitigate its effects.

Good Clinical Practice Points for Midwives and Maternity Services Working with Homeless Pregnant Women

- Open questions that specifically are related to the woman's current housing situation should be asked on at least four occasions: at booking, at 28 weeks, at 36 weeks and on postnatal discharge.
- A Duty to Refer referral should be made as soon as maternity services become aware that the woman is, or might be, homeless or threatened with homelessness.
- Try to arrange antenatal appointments at times that would be more appropriate if the woman is having to travel long distances, or consider carrying out routine antenatal appointments in the accommodation the woman is staying in.
- In view of the potential impact on the growth of the foetus and the increased risk of preterm labour, midwives should make every effort to work with the mother to closely monitor the wellbeing of the unborn baby.
- Routinely ask the woman at her antenatal appointments about her mental health and signposted or refer to the relevant support agencies.
- Midwives should discuss and offer referral into a nearby children's centre to obtain help from a family support worker and into any local third sector pregnancy support agencies.
- Ensure women who are eligible are assisted in applying for Healthy Start vouchers.
- Undertake an Early Help assessment for a coordinated multi-agency approach to support.
- Liaison with geographical health visitor between 24 and 26 weeks to ensure that the 28-week antenatal visit can be carried out to complete the health needs assessment.
- Offer and encourage parenting programmes such as the Solihull Approach* to support and enhance the parent-child relationship (*based on a model of containment, reciprocity and behaviour management using social learning theory).
- Carry out a home assessment visit at 36 weeks to assess suitability of accommodation, and liaise with local authority where concerns arise.
- Women and families who are identified with threatened or actual homelessness with no recourse to public funds should be referred to Children's Services, ideally before the birth of the baby so that assessments can begin and discharges are not delayed from hospital.
- Take into account the role that homelessness or adult social services may be able to play in order to avoid breaches in the mother's human rights if accommodation is not initially provided.
- Develop strong links and good working relationships with the local housing authority.

- Liaison with the local authority regarding a move into a more suitable property if the woman has been in a B&B accommodation for longer than the 6 weeks laid down in statute; the woman develops gestation diabetes and does not have access to kitchen facilities; or the woman is still in a B&B-type accommodation over 30 weeks gestation or at the time of the birth.
- Clear and effective liaison with out-of-area community midwives to ensure that midwifery care is seamless across hospital boundaries and county borders when women are accommodated outside of the Trust catchment area.
- Clear verbal handovers, ideally by way of a discharge planning meeting, to health visitors, GP's and any other professionals working with the family when maternity care comes to an end.

References

1. Ministry of Housing, Communities and Local Government. *Statutory homelessness and prevention and relief, July to September (Q3) 2017: England.* 2018. https://www.gov.uk/government/statistical-data-sets/live-tables-on-homelessness
2. Welsh Government. *Homelessness in Wales, 2017–18—Revised. SFR 63/2018(R).* Statistical First Release. 2018. https://gweddill.gov.wales/docs/statistics/2018/180801-homelessness-2017-18-revised-en.pdf
3. Fitzpatrick S, Pleace N. The statutory homelessness system in England: a fair and effective rights-based model. Hous Stud. 2012;27(2):232–51. https://doi.org/10.1080/02673037.2012.632622.
4. Walsh K, Harvey B. Family experiences of pathways into homelessness: the families perspective. Dublin: Housing Agency; 2015.
5. Homeless Link. Supporting women who are homeless. Briefing for homelessness services. London, Homeless Link; 2017.
6. Corston J. The Corston report. London: Crown Copyright; 2007.
7. Reeve K, Casey R, Goudie R. Homeless women: still being failed yet striving to survive. London: Crisis; 2006.
8. Fingfeld-Connett D. Becoming homeless, being homeless, and resolving homelessness among women. Issues Ment Health Nurs. 2010;31(7):461–9. https://doi.org/10.3109/01612840903586404.
9. Taylor Gaubatz K. Family homelessness in Britain: more than just a housing issue. J Child Poverty. 2001;7(1):3–22. https://doi.org/10.1080/10796120120038000.
10. Ministry of housing, communities and local government, rough sleeping strategy (London, 2018).
11. Sawtell M. Lives on hold: homeless families in temporary accommodation. London: Maternity Alliance; 2002.
12. Tischler V, Rademeyer A, Vostanis P. Mothers experiencing homelessness: mental health, support and social care needs. Health Soc Care Community. 2007;15(3):246–53. https://doi.org/10.1111/j.1365-2524.2006.00678.x.
13. Perlman S, Cowan B, Gewirtz A, Haskett M, Stokes L. Promoting positive parenting in the context of homelessness. Am J Orthopsychiatry. 2012;82(3):402–12. https://doi.org/10.1111/j.1939-0025.2012.01158.x.

14. Gültekin L, Brush BL, Baiardi JM, Kirk K, Van Maldeghem K. Voices from the street: exploring the realities of family homelessness. J Fam Nurs. 2014;20(4):390–414. https://doi.org/10.1177/1074840714548943.
15. Swick KJ, Williams R, Fields E. Parenting while being homeless. Early Child Educ J. 2014;42:397–403. https://doi.org/10.10007/s10643-013-0620-7.
16. Anthony ER, Vincent A, Shin Y. Parenting and child experiences in shelter: a qualitative study exploring the effect of homelessness on the parent-child relationship. Child Fam Soc Work. 2018;23:8–15. https://doi.org/10.1111/cfs.12376.
17. Shelter. Desperate to escape: the experiences of homeless families in emergency accommodation. London: Shelter; 2016.
18. Shelter. Summary: 'We've got no home': The experiences of homeless children in emergency accommodation. 2017. https://england.shelter.org.uk/__data/assets/pdf_file/0008/1471067/2017_Christmas_investigation_report.pdf
19. Reynolds L. The housing crisis generation: how many children are homeless in Britain? London: Shelter; 2018. https://england.shelter.org.uk/__data/assets/pdf_file/0004/1626466/The_housing_crisis_generation_-_Homeless_children_in_Britain.pdf
20. Fitzpatrick S, Christian J. Comparing homelessness research in the US and Britain. Eur J Hous Policy. 2006;6(3):313–33. https://doi.org/10.1080/14616710600973151.
21. Housing (England) Act 1996. Part VII: Homelessness.
22. FEANTSA. ETHOS –European Typology of Homelessness and housing exclusion. 2017. http://www.feantsa.org/download/ethos3742009790749358476.pdf
23. Legislation.gov.uk. Homelessness Reduction Act 2017. 2017. https://www.legislation.gov.uk/ukpga/2017/13/contents/enacted.
24. Homelessness (Review Procedure etc.) Regulations 2018 SI 2018/223.
25. Local Government Association. Duty to refer: an opportunity to cooperate to tackle homelessness. Advice for local housing authorities. London: Local Government Association; 2018.
26. Homelessness (Priority Need for Accommodation) (England) Order 2002
27. Ministry of Housing, Communities & Local Government. Homelessness code of guidance for local authorities. 2018. https://www.gov.uk/guidance/homelessness-code-of-guidance-for-local-authorities
28. https://www.gov.uk/evicting-tenants/section-21-and-section-8-notices
29. Wilson W, Barton C. Households in temporary accommodation (England). Briefing paper number 02110, 19 March 2019. London: House of Commons Library; 2019.
30. Bimpson E, Reeve K & Parr S. Homeless mothers: key research findings. Other. UK Collaborative Centre for Housing Evidence (CaCHE). 2020.
31. Thomas KA, So M. Lost in limbo: an exploratory study of homeless mothers' experiences and needs at emergency assistance hotels. Families Soc J Contemp Social Serv. 2016;97(2):12–131. https://doi.org/10.1606/1044-3894.2016.97.15.
32. The Homelessness (Suitability of Accommodation) (England) Order 2003 (SI 2003/3326).
33. Ministry of Housing, Communities and Local Government. Temporary accommodation live tables. 2018. https://www.gov.uk/government/statistical-data-sets/live-tables-on-homelessness#statutory-homelessness-live-tables
34. Jones H & Solicitors A. Webpage—B&B accommodation, skirting the '6 week rule'. 2018. https://www.hja.net/bb-accommodation-skirting-the-6-week-rule/
35. Homeless Link. Supporting people with no recourse to public funds (NRPF). Guidance for homelessness services. Homeless Link: London; 2020.
36. https://www.citizensadvice.org.uk/about-us/how-citizens-advice-works/media/press-releases/citizens-advice-reveals-nearly-14m-have-no-access-to-welfare-safety-net/
37. Immigration and Asylum Act 1999. London: The Stationary Office.
38. Nationality, Immigration and Asylum Act 2014. London: Crown Copyright.
39. Chartered institute of Housing. Refugees, asylum seekers and people with discretionary leave and humanitarian protection—webpage. 2020. https://www.housing-rights.info/02_2_Refugees.php

40. UK Visas & Immigration. A Home Office Guide to Living in Asylum Accommodation. https://assets.publishing.service.gov.uk/government/uploads/system/uploads/attachment_data/file/821324/Pack_A_-_English_-_Web.pdf
41. Feldman R. What price safe motherhood? Charging for NHS maternity care in England and its impact on migrant women. London: Maternity Action; 2018.
42. Allsopp J, Sigona N and Phillimore J. Poverty among refugees and asylum seekers in the UK: An evidence and policy review. 2014. http://www.birmingham.ac.uk/Documents/college-social-sciences/socialpolicy/iris/2014/working-paper-series/IRiS-WP-1-2014.pdf
43. Home Office & UK Visas and Immigration. National referral mechanism guidance: adult (England and Wales). 2020. https://www.gov.uk/government/publications/human-trafficking-victims-referral-and-assessment-forms/guidance-on-the-national-referral-mechanism-for-potential-adult-victims-of-modern-slavery-england-and-wales
44. Pillinger C, O'Doherty L & Bowen E. Migrant women's experiences of sexual and gender-based violence and help-seeking strategies (University of Coventry). 2017.
45. Home Office. Destitute domestic violence (DDV) concession. Version 1.0. 2018. https://assets.publishing.service.gov.uk/government/uploads/system/uploads/attachment_data/file/679269/victims-of-domestic-violence-and-abuse-DDV-concession-v1_0.pdf#:~:text=The%20DDV%20concession%20only%20applies%20to%20applicants%20who,the%20following%3A%20o%20British%20citizen%20o%20settled%20person.
46. Chartered Institute of Housing. Webpage—What is the habitual residence test? 2020. https://www.housing-rights.info/habitual-residence-test.php
47. Ministry of Housing, Communities & Local Government. Homelessness code of guidance for local authorities. 2020. https://www.gov.uk/guidance/homelessness-code-of-guidance-for-local-authorities/annex-1-the-habitual-residence-test
48. Department for Communities and Local Government. Statutory Homelessness and Prevention and Relief live tables: Table 774—Reason for Loss of last Settled Home. 2017. Online: DCLG. https://www.gov.uk/government/statistical-data-sets/live-tables-on-homelessness.
49. Saewyc EM. Influential life contexts and environments for out-of-home pregnant adolescents. J Holist Nurs. 2003;21(4):343–67. https://doi.org/10.1177/0898010103258607.
50. Smid M, Bourgois P, Auerswald CL. The challenge of pregnancy among homeless youth: reclaiming a lost opportunity. J Health Care Poor Underserved. 2010;21(2 Suppl):140–56. https://doi.org/10.1353/hpu.0.0318.
51. Berkum AV, Ouddshoorn A. Best practice guideline for ending Women's and Girl's homelessness. Canada: Women's Community House; 2015.
52. Fortin R, Jackson SF, Maher F, Moravac C. I WAS HERE: young mothers who have experienced homelessness use Photovoice and participatory qualitative analysis to demonstrate strengths and assets. Glob Health Promot. 2015;22(1):8–20. https://doi.org/10.1177/1757975914528960.
53. Leng G. The impact of homelessness on health. A guide for local authorities. London: Local Government Association; 2017.
54. Moore R. Coping with homelessness: an expectant mother's homeless pathway. Hous Care Support. 2014;17(3):142–50. https://doi.org/10.1108/HCS-02-2014-0002.
55. Finfgeld-Connett D. Becoming homeless, being homeless, and resolving homelessness among women. Issues Ment Health Nurs. 2010;31(7):461–9. https://doi.org/10.3109/01612840903586404.
56. Reynolds S. "You shouldn't have to feel you're pushing your pregnancy aside." A study of women's reflections on their experiences of becoming homeless during their pregnancy in the UK. [Unpublished master's dissertation] University of Hertfordshire. 2019.
57. Martin-Fernandez J, et al. Food insecurity in homeless families in the Paris Region (France): results from the ENFAMS survey. Int J Environ Res Public Health. 2018;15(3):420. https://doi.org/10.3390/ijerph15030420.
58. Dachner N, Tarasuk V. Homeless "squeegee kids": food insecurity and daily survival. Soc Sci Med. 2002;54:1039–49.
59. Killion CM. Special health care needs of homeless pregnant women. Adv Nurs Sci. 1995;18(2):44–56.

60. Hobel C, Culhane J. Role of psychosocial and nutritional stress on poor pregnancy outcome. J Nutr. 2003;133(5):1709S–17S. https://doi.org/10.1093/jn/133.5.1709S.
61. Dunkel-Schetter C, Glynn L. Stress in pregnancy: empirical evidence and theoretical issues to guide interdisciplinary researchers. In: Contrada R, Baum A, editors. The handbook of stress science. New York: Springer; 2010.
62. Stein JA, Lu MC, Gelberg L. Severity of homelessness and birth outcomes. Health Psychol. 2000;19(6):524–34.
63. Carrion BV, Earnshaw VA, Kershaw T, Lewis JB, Stasko EC, Tobin JN, Ickovics JR. Housing instability and birth weight among young urban mothers. J Urban Health. 2014;92(1):1–9. https://doi.org/10.1007/s11524-014-9913-4.
64. Cutts DB, Coleman S, Black MM, Chilton MM, Cook JT, de Cuba SE, Heeren TC, Meyers A, Sandel M, Casey PH, Frank DA. Homelessness during pregnancy: a unique, time-dependant risk factor of birth outcomes. Matern Child Health J. 2014;19(6):1276–83. https://doi.org/10.1007/s10995-014-1633-6.
65. Clarke A. Serious case review report child E. Kent: Kent Safeguarding Children Board; 2017. https://www.kscb.org.uk/__data/assets/pdf_file/0004/76558/20171107-Child-E-SCR-Final-Report.pdf
66. Little M, Shah R, Vermeulen MJ, Gorman A, Ray JG. Adverse perinatal outcomes associated with homelessness and substance use in pregnancy. Can Med Assoc J. 2005;173(6):615–8. https://doi.org/10.1503/cmaj.050406.
67. Richards R, Merrill RM, Baksh L. Health behaviours and infant health outcomes in homeless pregnant women in the United States. Pediatrics. 2011;128:438–46. https://doi.org/10.1542/peds.2010-349.
68. Hogg S, Haynes A, Baradon T, Cuthbert C. An unstable start. All babies count: spotlight on homelessness. London: NSPCC; 2015.
69. Easterbrook MA, Graham CA. Security of attachment and parenting: homeless and low-income housed mothers and infants. Am J Orthopsychiatry. 1999;69(3):337–46.
70. Moorman F. The impact of homelessness on young children: Building resilience through supportive early educational interventions. Master's Theses and Doctoral Dissertations. 2009, 230. http://commons.emich.edu/theses/230
71. Theodorou N, & Johnsen S. Homelessness and adverse childhood experience (ACE). Homeless in Europe. 2017, 4–7.
72. Brandon M, Sidebotham P, Bailey S, Belderson P, Hawley C, Ellis C, Megson M. New learning from serious case reviews: a two-year report for 2009–2011. London: Department for Education; 2012.
73. NSPCC. Housing services: learning from case reviews: Summary of risk factors and learning for improved practice around the housing sector. 2014. https://www.nspcc.org.uk/preventing-abuse/child-protection-system/case-reviews/learning/housing/
74. Johnson F & Trench S. Serious case review sofia. Local safeguarding Children Board. 2015. https://www.rbkc.gov.uk/pdf/Sofia%20SCR%20final%20report%20published%20Dec%202015.pdf
75. Birthrights and Birth Companions. Holding it all together: Understanding how far the human rights of woman facing disadvantage are respected during pregnancy, birth and postnatal care. London [online]. 2019.
76. Hunter B, Sanders J, Warren L. Exploring the public health role of midwives and maternity support workers: final report. Cardiff: Cardiff University; 2015.
77. Bloom KC, Bednarzyk MS, Devitt DL, Renault RA, Teaman V, van Loock DM. Barriers to prenatal care for homeless pregnant women. JOGNN. 2004;33:428–35. https://doi.org/10.1177/0884217504266677.
78. Semenya ML, Lane A. Prenatal care among women struggling with poverty or homelessness. Alta RN. 2006;62(7):16–7.
79. National Maternity Review. Better Births—Improving outcomes of maternity services in England—a Five Year Forward View for maternity care. 2016. http://tinyurl.com/NMR2016

80. The National Institute for Health and Care Excellence. Pregnancy and complex social factors: a model for service provision for pregnant women with complex social factors NICE guideline. Clinical Guidance [CG110]. 2010.
81. Royal College of Midwives. Duty to refer guidance for midwives on the homelessness reduction act (2017). London: Royal College of Midwives; 2019.
82. Department of Health. Safer maternity care: the National Maternity Safety Strategy – progress and next steps. London: Department of Health; 2017. https://assets.publishing.service.gov.uk/government/uploads/system/uploads/attachment_data/file/662969/Safer_maternity_care_-_progress_and_next_steps.pdf
83. NHS England. National maternity review. Better births: improving outcomes of maternity Services in England: a five year forward view for maternity care. . National Maternity Review London: NHS England; 2016. https://www.england.nhs.uk/wp-content/uploads/2016/02/national-maternity-review-report.pdf
84. Sandall J, Soltani H, Gates S, Shennan A, Devane D. Midwife-led continuity models versus other models of care for childbearing women. Cochrane Database Syst Rev. 2016;(4):CD004667. https://doi.org/10.1002/14651858.CD004667.pub5.
85. Rayment-Jones H, Silverio SA, Harris J, Harden A, Sandall J. Project 20: midwives' insight into continuity of care models for women with social risk factors: what works, for whom, in what circumstances, and how. Midwifery. 2020;84 https://doi.org/10.1016/j.midw.2020.102654.
86. Stringer M, Averbuch T, Brooks PM, Jemmott LS. Response to homeless childbearing women's health care learning needs. Clin Nurs Res. 2012;21(2):195–212. https://doi.org/10.1177/1054773811420769.
87. Legislation.gov.uk. Human Rights Act 1998. 1998. https://www.legislation.gov.uk/ukpga/1998/42/contents.
88. Equity and Homan Rights Commission. Webpage—Article 2: Right to life. 2018. https://www.equalityhumanrights.com/en/human-rights-act/article-2-right-life
89. Marmot M, Allen J, Goldblatt P, Boyce T, McNeish D, Grady M, Geddes I. Fair society, healthy lives: the Marmot review: strategic review of health inequalities in England post-2010. London: The Marmot Review; 2010. http://www.parliament.uk/documents/fair-society-healthy-lives-full-report.pdf
90. Department for Education. Working together to safeguard children. A guide to inter-agency working to safeguard and promote the welfare of children. London: Crown Copyright; 2018.
91. Hopper EK, Bassuk EL, Olivet J. Shelter from the storm: trauma-informed Care in Homelessness Service Settings. Open Health Serv Policy J. 2010;3:80–100. https://doi.org/10.2174/1874924001003010080.
92. Van Berkum A & Oudshoorn A. Best practice guideline for ending women's and girl's homelessness. 2015. https://www.deslibris.ca/ID/246858
93. Guarino KM. Trauma-informed care for families experiencing homelessness. In: Haskett M, Perlman S, Cowan B, editors. Supporting families experiencing homelessness. New York, NY: Springer; 2014. https://doi.org/10.1007/978-1-4614-8718-0_7.
94. Guarino K, Soares P, Konnath K, Clervil R, Bassuk E. Trauma-informed organizational toolkit. Rockville, MD: Center for Mental Health Services, Substance Abuse and Mental Health Services Administration, and the Daniels Fund, the National Child Traumatic Stress Network, and the W.K. Kellogg Foundation; 2009. www.homeless.samhsa.gov and www.familyhomelessness.org
95. Legislation.gov.uk. Localism Act 2011. 2011. https://www.legislation.gov.uk/ukpga/2011/20/contents/enacted.
96. NRPF network. Webpage—12. Victims of trafficking and modern slavery. 2020. http://guidance.nrpfnetwork.org.uk/reader/practice-guidance-adults/victims-of-trafficking-and-modern-slavery/#121-safeguarding-duty
97. Legislation.gov.uk. Care Act 2014. 2014. https://www.legislation.gov.uk/ukpga/2014/23/contents.
98. Children Act 1989. London: The Stationary Office.

99. Reis S. Migrant women and social security. A pre-budget briefing from the Women's Budget Group. 2020.
100. Legislation.gov.uk. Housing Act 1996. 1996. https://www.legislation.gov.uk/ukpga/1996/52/contents.
101. Equality and Human Rights Commission. Webpage—Article 3: Freedom from torture and inhuman or degrading treatment). 2018. https://www.equalityhumanrights.com/en/human-rights-act/article-3-freedom-torture-and-inhuman-or-degrading-treatment
102. Shelter. Webpage—Human rights challenges. 2019. https://england.shelter.org.uk/legal/homelessness_applications/challenging_la_decisions/human_rights_challenges
103. The Queen on the Application of Bernard v. London Borough of Enfield. EWHC 2282 (Admin). 2002. https://www.escr-net.org/caselaw/2015/queen-application-bernard-v-london-borough-enfield-2002-ewhc-2282-admin
104. Bowers J, Cheyne H. Reducing the length of postnatal hospital stay: implications for cost and quality of care. BMC Health Serv Res. 2015;16:16. https://doi.org/10.1186/s12913-015-1214-4.
105. Nursing and Midwifery Council. The Code. Professional standards of practice and behaviour for nurses, midwives and nursing associates. London: NMC; 2018.
106. Cardwell V & Wainwright L. Making Better Births a reality for women with multiple disadvantages. 2018. http://www.revolving-doors.org.uk/file/2333/download?token=P2z9dlAR
107. McLeish J, Redshaw M. Maternity experiences of mothers with multiple disadvantages in England: a qualitative study. Women Birth. 2019;32(2):178–84. https://doi.org/10.1016/j.wombi.2018.05.009.
108. NMC. Standards of proficiency for midwives. London: RCM; 2019.

Violence and Abuse in Pregnancy

7

Celia Wildeman

Abstract

Domestic violence and abuse has been known to occur for centuries. It has a catastrophic effect on society and affects women from physical, social, psychological and financial perspectives. Evidence suggests that violence can be initiated or escalated in pregnancy, and this has serious consequences for the safety of women and babies and care provision. Current research suggests that intervention is necessary to reduce the impact on family health and social wellbeing. The midwife has a significant role in ensuring that lasting and meaningful change occur.

Keywords

Violence · Abuse · Family · Midwives · Collaboration

7.1   Introduction

This chapter aims to promote and enhance confidence of midwives and student midwives when working with women who are in abusive relationships. Its purposes are to enable midwives to become more aware of the key communication elements: verbal and non-verbal cues that women might exhibit and indications to the negative treatment they endure. It will suggest the language that best facilitates disclosure, trust and respect by providing examples of best midwifery practice. It also aims to persuade midwives to be reflective in their practice to enable learning and change to occur.

C. Wildeman (✉)
School of Health and Social Work, University of Hertfordshire, Hatfield, UK
e-mail: c.wildeman@herts.ac.uk

© Springer Nature Switzerland AG 2021
L. Abbott (ed.), *Complex Social Issues and the Perinatal Woman*,
https://doi.org/10.1007/978-3-030-58085-8_7

Coming from a position of counselling women therapeutically for over 30 years, it is clear that violence and abuse in an intimate relationship devastates family's lives. This view has been expressed repeatedly by various authorities and agencies that deal with the challenges of this issue. The World Health Organization expressed the view that violence against women by an intimate partner is an important public health and human rights issue [1]. It is a well-known fact that violence and abuse can occur at any time in a relationship, but for some women, it is initiated or escalated during pregnancy [2]. Violence and abuse of pregnant and newly birthed women by an intimate partner is a complex issue because of the individual nature of its manifestation. Clearly, this has serious consequences not only for the woman but for the foetus and the family as a whole. It therefore requires the professional to be aware of the inverted nature of the phenomenon. Midwives are in a privileged position to intervene so as to prevent and reduce catastrophe from happening. However, currently, some midwives do not appear to feel able to deal with the complexity of domestic violence and abuse (DV and DA) [3]. This has created a gap in knowledge and practice [4].

7.2   Definition

According to the National Institute for Health and Care Excellence (NICE) [5], the term domestic violence and abuse is used to mean:

> *Any incident or pattern of incidents of controlling behavior, violence or abuse between those 16 years or over who are family members or who are or have been intimate partners.*

This includes psychological, physical, sexual, financial and emotional abuse. It also includes honour-based violence and forced marriage. Women's Aid [6], an organisation at the forefront of this issue, acknowledges the psychological, physical, sexual and financial aspects of domestic abuse and extended these unwelcomed behaviours of coercive and controlling behaviour. The elements of cohesion and control are useful in guiding midwives when identification and intervention are considered necessary. Mayhill (2015) found that women are far more likely than men to be victims of abuse that involves ongoing degradation and frightening threats—two key elements of coercive control [7]. Domestic violence and abuse is not a new concept. It has been described since biblical times, and indeed it has been reputed that the rule of thumb law to execute spousal abuse can be traced as far back as 1782, the year that James Gillray published Judge Thumb [8]. However, the prevalence and catastrophic effects have become increasingly evident over the recent years [9, 10]. This has resulted in Department of Health and Social Care publications and guidelines, acknowledging and informing professionals including midwives that they must be willing and able to respond to the needs of pregnant women who are experiencing violence and abuse in their relationships. Key principles and actions for professional guidance are zero tolerance by respecting the right to live without violence and abuse in the family, acting immediately to disclosure and responding to risk, ensuring child safety is paramount and considering the rights of the child to live safely, ensuring adult safety is a priority, applying sensitivity and being cautious of when to share information.

7.3   Facts and Figures

In 2016, Woodhouse and Dempsey stated that 1.3 million of women (8.2%) [7] were affected by domestic violence and abuse. This figure is believed to be an underestimate due to under-reporting in health and social care research studies, to the police and to other support services. Currently, six to eight women died at the hands of a violent partner which was a substantial increase [11]. One third of children witnessing domestic violence also experience other forms of abuse [12]. 130,000 live in households with high risk of domestic abuse and are more likely to have behavioural and emotional problems as a consequence [13]. There was an 85% increase in domestic violence in London, 230 cases each day [14]. Indeed, this year, the Government has appointed a commissioner for domestic violence who will monitor and put in place strategies to deal with domestic violence and abuse [15].

Women need courage and confidence to disclose domestic violence and abuse [3]. On average, a woman will experience 35 assaults before she will report it to the police or any of the support services [16]. Two women a week are killed by their current or former partner, and women aged 16–25 are at the highest risk [17]. These stark statistics should motivate the midwife to intervene by having the knowledge and practical expertise gained through the attendance at in-service sessions, conferences, workshops and keeping a reflexive diary.

Reflection

Consider conducting an antenatal interview with a very young woman, her partner and her 2-year-old daughter. The woman looks anxious, hesitant and nervous. Her partner is answering most of the questions directed to the woman. You have become consciously aware of this, and your curiosity has heightened. Do you interrupt the interview, or do you continue to ask her questions relevant to her antenatal appointment? Interrupting the interview could cause her great distress but on the other hand could portray care and concern however prolonging the time available. There is also the issue of the presence of her partner who has been making numerous attempts to intervene in the discussion. How would you manage this scenario without putting the woman and her child at risk?

Possible Solution

In this scenario, the midwife has a responsibility to ensure that the woman's physical and emotional safety are addressed. It would be prudent to reveal her concerns in a sensitive and empathetic manner away from the partner. Consider how best you could do this? It is important to trust the woman's response as this is an important attribute to portray. Fear of the consequences of her response, for example, what her partner might do/say or what the authorities might do, could prevent her from saying the true circumstances of her situation. Building a trusting relationship with her and good record-keeping and following the nursing and midwifery professional standards [18]—will all contribute to the quality of the interaction. It is also crucial to be aware that she could be in danger if she is not discretely protected as her partner is present.

7.4 Government Guidance

The Department of Health [19] again advised health professionals to routinely ask women about violence and abuse in their relationships. It recommended the development of local guidelines for referral to multidisciplinary teams. The National Institute for Health and Care Excellence [17] also supports the development of such guidelines. It states that local policies should include clear referral pathways, sources of support, information regarding safety and how to plan follow-up care. There are still many National Health Service Trusts that do not have a functional local protocol or guidelines [20], and midwife intervention can therefore be problematic without the appropriate pathways to support her/him.

Understanding the elements of cohesion and control domestic abuse should guide midwives when identification and intervention in cases of domestic abuse are considered necessary. Keeling and Fisher [21] noted low rates of identification of domestic violence in healthcare settings as the choice to disclose domestic violence is very complex. Indeed, midwives seem hesitant to ask the question of whether pregnant women are being abused. Some of the reasons identified are lack of confidence and uncertainty about referral procedures [15] but also that the midwife herself may be a survivor of abuse or violence.

7.4.1 Consider this Scenario of a Midwife Conducting a Postnatal Examination

Midwife Smith noticed that Jenny is overly subdued, not giving her eye contact as she usually did and avoiding responding to questions about her wellbeing. At a ward meeting later that day, the midwife expressed her concern about Jenny, and a general discussion ensued. The issue of possible domestic abuse was suggested as one of the team remembered that Jenny's partner was verbally abusive to her the previous evening. Jenny's midwife decided to re-visit the situation by having a private discussion with Jenny to explore her social and psychological care needs.

If midwives are going to make intervention progress, it is important that they understand different family values and how the professional can work with different family characteristics. For example, some families may consider that it is more important to keep their experience private, and the midwife may be considered to be an intruder. In this situation, the midwife would need to use knowledge, skill and diplomacy to persuade Jenny that she respects her views and decisions and that she is nonetheless available for advice and support unconditionally. It would be wise not to adopt the "all-knowing" professional stance as this has been demonstrated to alienate the woman and her family [3]. Indeed, these two aspects have been repeatedly cited by midwives and were dominantly named in a small-scale research project carried out as part of a Masters in Practice-Based Research Degree. The research method utilized a questionnaire with semi-structured tape-recorded interviews and a focus group [3]. Midwives and student midwives were questioned about them asking pregnant women routinely about violence and abuse in their intimate relationships. Invariably, the reply was clothed in lack of education and training to be able to work in a confident and knowledgeable way. The midwives admitted that they though they were willing, they did not feel confident to ask the question: *What if the woman gave a positive response? It could open a can of worms, and what would I then do?* The students lamented that they did not feel they received the guidance in practice that would enable them to feel confident to ask the question.

Current evidence suggests that midwives acknowledge their crucial role in identifying and managing domestic violence and abuse. Their unpreparedness appears to be based on various barriers that need to be overcome through education, training and support. At the centre of these obstacles is the need to implement basic university education on the subject and provision of specific professional training [3]. This education process should begin with curriculum planning and innovative integration of the issue of domestic violence and coercion into the academic and professional practice programme.

Midwives are in a unique position to offer support to women facing the challenges of domestic violence. Indeed, O'Reilly, Beale and Gillies [22] advise that pregnancy offers a unique opportunity to identify women who are experiencing domestic abuse. Additionally, the Nursing and Midwifery Council [23] and the Midwives Rules and Standards [24] suggest that "a midwife should enable the woman to make decisions about her care based on her individual needs by discussing matters fully with her" (p 18). The issue of domestic violence and abuse is a professional duty and responsibility, and midwives remain accountable for their actions and omissions.

There must be the quality and quantity of support and guidance to ensure that long-term and long-lasting positive change results from the midwife's involvement. Midwives' intervention must be safe for them and for women. Wright [25] is of the view that lack of training and clear protocols is the root cause of breakdown of many healthcare providers not being able to evaluate and confirm the usefulness and effectiveness of intervention strategies. Having the evidence that intervention is valuable and essential is important as embedding routine enquiry into routine midwifery practice raises women's expectations of care, and this can be realised. It also has positive implications for the development of midwifery practice.

Midwives however motivated and committed cannot work on their own to promote durable change. There is evidence that demonstrates best practice is achieved when domestic violence and abuse is tackled in a multi-professional way [26]. This way of working is supported by the Department of Health [26], Her Majesty's Government [27], and other agencies. It is useful to be aware of the tension between confidentiality and information sharing (Department of Health, 28). A gatekeeper's role ensures that the individual's personal records are divulged only as is necessary. Multi-agency victim-focused conferences are an example of where and how sensitive information is shared by professionals (DoH) [29] and highest risk cases of domestic abuse are so treated. A safety plan for each victim is created. Current general data protection (2018) rules and regulations must be in place [30]. Data protection, GDPR and privacy of the individual must also be adhered to—the Caldicott Guardian Principles protect data kept about individuals, preventing identification of an individual unless other information kept separately is sought.

7.5   The Role of the Midwife

The National Institute for Health and Care Excellence (NICE) [31] stated that the human and economic effects of domestic violence and abuse are so vast that even marginal interventions are cost-effective. It emphasised that heterosexual women experience more physical assaults and other violence, more repeated and severe violence, much more sexual violence, more cohesive control, more injuries and an increased fear of their partner [31]. Midwives are in a strategic position to significantly influence positive change in a pregnant woman's health and also have a major role to protect and improve the health of pregnant women through education and health promotion [19]. The intimate nature of the midwife/woman relationship and the need of the woman to protect her unborn child are factors associated with increased disclosure of domestic abuse during pregnancy. The nature of the midwife's role and the intimacy of the relationship between the woman and her midwife can be a difficult-to-broach sensitive subject described as challenging and complicated [23].

The Department of Health [32] acknowledges that because of her role, the midwife is often one of the first professionals to become aware of domestic violence and abuse issues within the family. Midwives have a significant part to play by advocating, championing and supporting affected women. The long-lasting and negative impact across a wide range of health, social, emotional and intellectual development of the child and young person and indeed the family unit reinforces the need for midwives to exercise professional judgement at all times [31].

It is clearly documented that midwives must assert themselves and routinely ask pregnant women about violence and abuse in their relationships [31, 17]. Advocating for women is one important way of demonstrating the concept of being "with woman" [33]. The Department of Health acknowledges and recognises the factors that may indicate domestic violence and abuse. It describes steps that will ensure appropriate support and referral of those affected when this is necessary. The elements of best practice, key information and resources for learning are all indicated in its guidelines [31]. Midwives should be cognisant of the facts if they are going to be able to advocate and support women in a respectful and knowledgeable manner. However, the emotional burden of dealing with this complex and sensitive issue for midwives appears to be under-identified and under-addressed [3, 31]. Midwifery is a female-dominated profession, and therefore midwives will be represented in this statistic further complicating the issue by potentially triggering negative feelings about addressing domestic abuse. The evidence supports the fact that being a midwife with a personal history of domestic abuse may be a factor associated with reluctance of midwives to enquire about domestic abuse [32].

Following key components of effective practice (Department of Health and Social Care guidance [16] will enable somewhere to enabling success in this area. Guidance includes:

- Never assume that someone else is addressing the domestic violence and abuse issues.
- It is not the professional's role to comment on or encourage the woman to leave her partner.
- Enquire sensitively.
- Create an opportunity providing a quiet environment where confidentiality can be assured for the woman to talk about her experiences.
- Be familiar with and give relevant information, if non-disclosure but you suspect domestic abuse is an issue.
- Accept the woman's decision not to disclose any information, but offer other opportunities, focus on safety and ensure proper documentation.
- Be familiar with local child protection procedures and use as appropriate.
- Share information appropriately.
- Use professional interpreters, not family members, friends or children, and be aware of your own safety needs.
- At every visit, listen, assess, action and document.

In 2018 [34], the Royal College of Midwives clearly suggested that midwives should ask women about domestic abuse. In response, it is apparent that this is still not routinely done [35] and that indeed not all National Health Service (NHS) Trusts have clear functional guidelines that support their staff in this complex and sensitive aspect of service provision [36].

The National Institute for Health and Care Excellence [17] and the Department of Health [16] both support the view that women should be routinely asked about violence and abuse in their relationships. Clearly, this is a controversial issue and one that may not always be easy to implement in practice.

The quality of the relationship women builds with midwives [37] and being supported not to feel ashamed and not to self-blame will all help to encourage women to disclose violence and abuse. Midwives should be careful to ask questions in a sensitive and meaningful way, for example, ascertaining information from the woman's own perspective:

- How does the violence affect you?
- Who else in the family is affected?
- What helps you to cope?
- Where do you best get support and who or where does it come from?

These kinds of questions enable the woman to reflect on her situation and at the same time consider potential solutions to her problem.

7.6   Collaborative Working

Working collaboratively in a multi-professional context requires midwives and allied health professionals to have knowledge, skills, the right attitude and confidence to respond appropriately to positive disclosure [31]. The quality of resourcefulness for this model of working is recognised by like-minded agencies and researchers, for example, Martha et al. [38]. In their study of midwives' experiences of pregnant women victims of domestic abuse, they found that an inter-disciplinary approach was an important resource. However, midwives must be alert to the need to continue to search for robust evidence on the effectiveness of referral to the multi-professional team, before embracing a collaborative approach. This is because including another agency changes the dynamics and may negatively affect the midwife/woman relationship. The overall view is that a multi-professional collaborative approach results in improved disclosure by pregnant women about domestic violence [39]. Indeed, the acceptability of pregnant women to being asked routinely about violence and abuse in their intimate relationship is positive. Women want to be asked about their intimate relationships as this is an important area of their lives.

7.7   Cultural Issues and the Midwifery Role

The issue of cultural diversity and how this may impact on the willingness of women to disclose must be considered by the midwife. Additionally, the woman's age, ethnic group and social and educational status all contribute to the interactive exchange between woman and midwife. According to the Royal College of Midwives [24], 80% of women in abusive relationships sought help at least once, and it took them 7–8 visits before disclosures of abuse were made. These figures suggest that routine questioning is necessary, even essential to disclosure. Stonard and Whapples [32] state that 92% of midwives agree that they had a major part to play in the screening of domestic abuse. However, a significant but lower number, 28%, reported that they raised the issue when they had performed booking appointments. Clearly, there is tension between what midwives believe they should be doing and what they did. Adding language barriers and learning difficulties compounds the situation particularly in the context of cultural diversity.

7.8 Suggested Strategy to Asking Women about Domestic Abuse

It is indeed important for midwives to carry out an antenatal booking, confidently asking pregnant women routinely about violence and abuse, but they have repeatedly stated that they need professional guidance and practice in how to proceed with this strategy. The following are examples of how midwives might ask pregnant women about violent and abusive episodes in their intimate relationships:

1. Update by reading, discussing with the multidisciplinary team, ward meetings, midwifery education team and any other available forum or platform. Acquaint yourself with the current literature and research evidence. These actions are significant to the development of confidence and the readiness to confront this sensitive issue.
2. The questioning environment should be carefully considered. Discussions with student midwives and midwives [3] suggest that they find the often inappropriateness of the care environment to be daunting when voicing sensitive questions. It is important that the environment is calm, welcoming, private and confidential. For many of these women, trust is an issue, and the quality of the place in which the question is asked is vitally important. It is helpful to be direct, using language that is easily understood, for example:
   - *We ask all pregnant women about violence and abuse in their intimate relationship.*
   - *Have you experienced physical violence, emotional abuse or any other forms of abuse or bad treatment in your intimate relationship?*
   - *Tell me how you would describe your relationship?*
        The midwife must be prepared to listen actively and patiently and to observe non-verbal clues that the woman may be displaying. This is important so that the midwife can assess what the woman is saying and not saying. Any doubt should be checked and clarified. Assumptions should be avoided. The midwife's awareness of her own verbal as well as her non-verbal communication skills will facilitate congruence and authenticity which are key components of relating sensitively to the woman. The woman will be checking for these signals from the midwife. Genuineness goes a long way and will enable the woman to disclose the true nature of her intimate relationship.
3. Ending the conversation is equally important. The woman must be reassured that any decision is made in her best interest, that the midwife has heard and understood her situation and that a plan of care is mutually agreed. This includes any

referral to the multidisciplinary team. Even when there is safeguarding issues, this should be as far as possible discussed in a sensitive and honest way.

4. The plan of care should consist of follow-up strategies. The most appropriate care provider to monitor the woman's situation and to keep the multi-disciplinary team informed should be decided.

There are many reasons why midwives say they do not intervene. These reasons are clearly valid and should be taken seriously as safety for both the midwife and woman is paramount. Repeatedly, midwives identify real factors that impact on them intervening. One significant aspect is the presence of the woman's partner at the antenatal appointment [3, 17]. There are various confidential and sensitive ways to facilitate this process. Consider your local midwifery care environment and the facilities you have that can be utilized to deal with the possible presence of the woman's partner. This is a useful opportunity to reflect on your professional practice.

This scenario should provide both knowledge and practice for the midwife to confidently and professionally manage domestic violence and abuse that may occur in the lives of pregnant women and after the birth of the baby.

Jessica Williams has been married to John Williams for 4 years. They have one son David, aged 2. Jessica is now 4 months pregnant. John is out of work and has started drinking alcohol heavily. They argue continually, and John has been verbally and physically abusive. Jessica has arrived for her first antenatal appointment (one of numerous requests), and John is present. On reading her obstetric notes, you noticed that she has ignored all previous invitations to attend the antenatal clinic. During discussions, she disclosed that she rarely goes out and apologised for missing her previous appointments. She refers to John before she responds to the required antenatal history questions, and he looked intensely on her, and non-verbal clues suggested that she was uncomfortable with the situation. You realised that you needed to speak to Jessica on her own but are unsure about the safest way to do so without making John suspicious.

- **How would you deal with the situation?**
- **Who will you inform?**
- **What records will you document?**
- **How will your records be stored?**
- **How do you plan to monitor and review Jessica's situation?**

7.8.1   How Would you Deal with the Situation?

There are a number of approaches to this situation. As the midwife responsible for Jessica's care you could, for example, request a specimen of urine as a way of getting her away from John's scrutiny. Once she is made psychologically and physically comfortable, explain that you have noticed that she is uncomfortable in John's presence. Describe confidentiality issues with regard to safeguarding, and ask the question honestly and openly, for example, "are you being hurt at home?" Listen actively to her verbal response, and observe her non-verbal clues.

7.8.2   Who Will you Inform?

It is important that any professional guidelines and protocols are followed. They are there to inform the midwife, to enhance her /his confidence and to protect her/him and the woman. Inform your senior midwife/manager of Jessica's situation as soon as practically possible.

7.8.3   What Records Will you Document?

It is mandatory to have an accurate record of Jessica's situation. On examination, arrangements can be made for photographs to be taken if appropriate and with her consent. These are as previously exposed part of record-keeping. Comprehensive records are time-consuming but crucial to the management of Jessica's care. It is important to document correct date and time, what the concerns are, any information given by Jessica, what action if any that has been taken, who has been informed and the observed attitude of her partner.

7.8.4   How Will your Records be Stored?

Currently, most National Health Service (NHS) Trusts operate a client-held system for the woman's records. In Jessica's situation, this can put her in extreme danger of escalation of the abused. It is important that an agreed system is in operation, for example, a coding system. This will enable information to be gathered and stored in the most effective way. As with confidential records, her client notes should be kept secure, and other professional staff should know how to retrieve them so that continuity and safety are assured.

7.8.5 How Do you Plan to Monitor and Review Jessica's Situation?

As part of quality, woman-centred care monitoring and review are essential. Domestic violence and abuse is, as previously exposed, a complex issue. The midwife cannot manage this on her own. It requires a multi-professional team to ensure that Jessica's vital needs are achieved. Referral to the team as appropriate should be organized by the midwife. It is important to have a coherent plan and to re-visit it as often as is necessary. In this situation, the midwife may need to decide if it is safe for Jessica to return home, and if not the relevant professional personnel would be informed including any safeguarding issues as is appropriate. Ensure that Julia has a follow-up appointment for the clinic.

Above is a suggested guide only. The midwife needs to draw on her professional experience, ethical belief system, knowledge and degree of confidence. The Nursing and Midwifery Code of Ethics [12] should be utilized so as to act in the best interest of her clients.

7.9 Conclusion

This chapter has explored issues relating to domestic violence and the childbearing woman. Drawing upon best practice and current research evidence, suggestions have been made for professional practice and reflection. Domestic violence and abuse is a complex social and psychological public health issue and is becoming increasingly so for the twenty-first century. Midwives have a pivotal role to play in advocating for governmental, professional and social care strategies that will enhance the protection of women and families from this potentially catastrophic issue.

References

1. World Health Organization. *Violence against women: intimate partner and sexual violence against women.* Fact sheet 239. Geneva: WHO. Violence WHO; 2014.
2. Wakoma TT, Jampala L, Bexhill H, Gutheri K, Lindow S. Violence in women requesting a termination of pregnancy and those attending the antenatal clinic. Sex Health. 2014;D01. 10111/1471-052812609
3. Wildeman C. An investigation into the difficulties and barriers midwives face in asking pregnant and newly delivered women about partner violence and abuse. University of Hertfordshire; 2018. Unpublished
4. National Institute for Health and Care Excellence (NICE). Domestic violence and abuse Quality standard [QS116] 2016 [cited 2021 Mar 28]. https://www.nice.org.uk/guidance/qs116.
5. Women's Aid, What is domestic violence. London: Women's Aid; 2010.
6. Woodhouse J & Dempsey N. House of Commons Library. *Briefing paper* (6337). House of Commons 2016.
7. Mayhill A. Measuring coercive control: what can we learn from national population surveys? Sage. 2015;21(3):355–75.
8. British Broadcasting Corporation 1. *Breakfast Programme.* August 19: BBC 2019.

9. Radford L. Child abuse and neglect in the United Kingdom today. London: National Society for the Prevention of cruelty to children (NSPCC); 2011.
10. National Society for the Prevention of Cruelty to Children. Effects of child abuse. London: NSPCC; 2018.
11. BBC. *Breakfast Programme.* 2019.
12. Nursing and Midwifery Council. Standards of professional ethics and behavior. London: NMC; 2015.
13. Forster E. *Maternal violence: an english family history.* 1660–1857. Cambridge: University Press; 2005.
14. Stonyard J, Whapples E. Domestic violence in pregnancy, midwives and routine questioning. The Practicing Midwjfe. 2016;19(1):26–9.
15. Salmon D, Baird K, White P. Women's views and experiences of antenatal enquiry for domestic abuse during pregnancy. Health Expect. 2013;18:867–78.
16. Department of Health and Social Care. Guidance for health professionals on domestic violence. London: Department of Health; 2013.
17. National Institute for Health and Care Excellence (NICE). *Pregnancy and complex social factors: a model for service provision for pregnant women with complex social factors.* Clinical guidelines 110. London: Collaborating Centre for Women and Children's Health; 2010.
18. Department of Health. Domestic violence—a resource manual for health care professionals. HMSO: DOH; 2000.
19. Department of Health. Guidance for health professionals on domestic violence. London: DOH; 2013.
20. Lenegham S, Sinclair M, Gillen P. Domestic abuse in pregnancy: I'm more used to unhealthy relationships so don't have a clue about healthy relationships. Evidence based Midwifery. 2015;13(4):120–5.
21. Keeling J, Fisher T. Health professionals responses to women's disclosure of domestic violence. J Interpers Violence. 2015;30(13):2363–78.
22. O'Rielly R, Beale B, Gillies D. Screening and intervention for domestic violence during pregnancy care: a systematic review. Trauma Violence Abuse. 2010;11(4):190–201.
23. Nursing and Midwifery Council. Definition of a midwife. London: NMC; 2010.
24. Nursing and Midwifery Council. Midwives rules and standards. London: NMC; 2004.
25. Wright L. Asking about domestic violence. Br J Nurs. 2003;11(4):199–202.
26. Department of Health. Responding to domestic abuse—a handbook for health professionals. London: DOH; 2017.
27. Her Majesty's Government (2016). Ending violence against women and girls. Strategy 2016–2020. London: HMSO.
28. National Institute for Health and Care Excellence. Violence and abuse, multi-agency working. (PW 50). London: NICE; 2014.
29. Department of Health. *Striking the balance, practical guidance on the application of the Caldecott Guidance Principles to domestic violence and multi-agency* (MARACS). London: DOH; 2012.
30. General data protection Rules. E U 2016/679. https//ec.europa.eu, 2018.
31. Harkness M, Lindohf J. Talking about domestic abuse during pregnancy. The Practicing Midwife. 2019:9–13.
32. Buck L, Collins S. Why don't midwives ask about domestic abuse? Br J Midwifery. 2007;15:753–7.
33. Office of National Statistics. Crime survey for England and Wales. London: ONS; 2015.
34. Royal College of Midwives. Position paper. London: RCM; 2018.
35. Price S, Baird K. Does routine antenatal enquiry lead to an increase rate of disclosure of domestic violence in pregnancy? Bristol: The Bristol Pregnancy and Domestic Violence Programme; 2007.
36. Baird K Salmon D White P. *A five year follow-up study of the British Pregnancy and domestic violence programme to promote routine antenatal enquiry for domestic violence at North Bristol University of West England.* 2011. ISBN: 978–1- 86-643-460-0.

37. United Nations International Children Emergency Fund. Hidden in plain sight: a statistical analysis of violence against children. New York: UNICEF; 2014. ISBN 928-92-806-98. Quality of Midwife/woman relationship
38. Martha MME, Respoli A, Persico G, Franca Z. Domestic violence during pregnancy—midwives experience. Midwifery. 2015;31:498–504.
39. Feder G, Agrew-davies, Baird K, Dunne D, Eldridge S, Griffiths C. Identification and referral to improve safety (IRIS) of women experiencing domestic violence. Lancet. 2011;378(9805):1788–95.

Perinatal Women in Prison

8

Laura Abbott

Abstract

It is understood that many women who end up in the criminal justice system are from extremely disadvantaged backgrounds. These may include being survivors of sexual abuse and neglect in childhood, being in the care of the local authority, being homeless, being survivors of domestic violence and misusing drugs and alcohol. It is known that a high proportion of women in prison suffer from mental ill health and complex post-traumatic stress disorder. This group of women is at particularly high risk of health complications in pregnancy. The following chapter reflects the experience of pregnant women in prison, considering their maternity care needs for each trimester and during the post-natal period. The chapter gives an overview of the current research undertaken, considering the demographics and characteristics of women who may become incarcerated and their health outcomes and the psychological impact of imprisonment. Vignettes illuminate the experiences of women in relation to human rights, toxic stress, the fear of going into labour at night, the shame experienced and the impact of being separated from their baby. Throughout the chapter, the reader is asked to consider their professional responsibilities and to look at their own unconscious bias when caring for the pregnant prisoner.

Keywords

Prison · Pregnancy · Institutions · Qualitative research · Human rights

L. Abbott (✉)
Department of Allied Health and Midwifery, University of Hertfordshire, Hatfield, Hertfordshire, UK
e-mail: l.abbott@herts.ac.uk

© Springer Nature Switzerland AG 2021
L. Abbott (ed.), *Complex Social Issues and the Perinatal Woman*,
https://doi.org/10.1007/978-3-030-58085-8_8

Key Learning Points
By the end of this chapter, readers will:

- Understand the social, psychological and economic background of women in prison
- Consider the prison environment and how this may impact upon the perinatal woman
- Understand the specific needs of the perinatal woman in prison and how these may differ from women in the community
- Consider how care can be delivered to enhance outcomes for women and their babies
- Consider interventions for women in prison in the context of midwifery and other universal services
- Consider individual needs in differing circumstances, e.g. the woman who is being separated from her baby or the woman who maintains the bond with her baby on an MBU

Vignette
"I was handcuffed in the hospital and even if I wanted to run off I couldn't … I am pregnant and it's such a (sighs) degrading experience and I know they have got procedures to follow but it wasn't even like the short handcuffs it was the ones with long chains on which are heavy … it is quite upsetting especially having a male officer there because I think the 1st man to see the scan of my unborn baby should be the father, not an officer." (Gemma)

8.1 Background

Women in prison make up roughly 2–10% of the global incarcerated population, with the USA having the greatest number of imprisoned women at 12% per 100,000 of the national population [1]. The UK has the highest prisoner population in the European Union with England and Wales having one of the highest figures at 6.7% per 100,000 of the national population [2]. In the UK, numbers of pregnant women are not routinely collated, but estimations suggest that 6–7% of the female prison population are at varying stages of pregnancy and approximately 100 babies are born to incarcerated women each year [3–7].

8.2 Women in Prison (UK)

The numbers of women held in UK prisons have been growing over the past 20 years [8]. There are currently 12 women's prisons in the UK and 6 Mother and Baby Units

(MBU[1]) attached with 54 places available for mothers with their babies up to the approximate age of 18 months old (ibid). Women prisoners may be held as one of four security categories: Category A, Restricted Status, Closed conditions or Open conditions.[2] Ten of the female estates in the UK are closed prisons,[3] holding women who are categorised as A, restricted status and closed conditions. There are two open prisons[4] (D Category) where women are sentenced if they meet the requirements or prior to resettlement into the community.

8.3   Demographics of Female Prisoners

A considerable number of women in prison have themselves been victims of crime and often have multiple complex needs and difficult lives. Current statistics suggest that:

- 46% have violent partners.
- 53% may have suffered sexual abuse and rape.
- 50% women have endured domestic violence.
- 66% are substance abusers.
- 31% spent time in care as a child.
- 80% of women suffer some form of mental health disorder [6, 9–12].

Most women enter the system already pregnant, and this is often revealed at initial health checks on reception to prison [10, 13]. However, exact numbers are not known or whether their pregnancies are coincidental or intentional [4].

8.4   Rights and Entitlements of the Perinatal Woman in Prison

The United Nations (UN) Bangkok Rules [14] recommend that women in prison should be given gender-specific care, and in the UK, the Council of Europe [15] states that every prisoner should receive healthcare equivalence. Article 3 of the

---

[1] A mother and baby unit places women who have successfully gained a place, with their babies up to 18 months of age.

[2] **Category A prisoners** are deemed the most dangerous prisoners who require the strictest security conditions. **Restricted status** is any woman on remand or sentenced who poses a serious risk to public safety. **Closed conditions** are for women who are too substantial a risk for open conditions although require less security. **Open conditions** are women who can be trusted and are a minimal risk to the public. PSI 39/2011

[3] A closed prison is maximum security holding Category A, restricted status, closed conditions and remand prisoners.

[4] An open prison is a minimum-security prison where women can attend outside work and are trusted with minimal supervision.

Human Rights Act [16]⁵ have a strong, legal basis in the UK with all women having the right to make decisions about her body during pregnancy with respectful treatment [17]. Article 8 protects the right to private life and ensures "choice" has a legal basis with the principle of dignity a priority. Economically, accountability for funding lies with the Department of Health (DH) and the Strategic Health Authority (SHA). Presently, private healthcare providers deliver prison healthcare for 21 prisons in England and Wales [18]. There is no known requirement for midwives to be located permanently in healthcare departments in prison; however, midwives do visit to provide antenatal and post-natal care in prison [7]. In one UK prison, a specialist midwife for the criminal justice system has a substantive role coordinating the care for all perinatal women and women who have given birth in the previous 12 months. The post was developed in response to the suicide of Michelle Barnes 5 days following the birth of her third baby [19], and there are calls for specialist midwives to coordinate care in all UK prisons [20]. More recently, the UK media have reported on concerns that pregnant women had given birth in their prison cells without access to a midwife [21], and the death of a newborn baby in prison has prompted widespread condemnations [22].

The UK Prison Service details guidance for the treatment of perinatal women in prison within a Prison Service Order (PSO).⁶ The guidance directs the prison service to make adequate provisions for women, e.g. women wishing to breastfeed their babies, advises suitable nutrition and adequate rest and suggests that careful planning should take place when women are being separated from their babies due to the risk to her mental health. The Royal College of Midwives [23] recommends that all pregnant prisoners should receive the same quality of care as if they were on the outside and has issued guidance in relation to incarcerated pregnant women and new mothers. There is no specific direction from organisations such as the National Institute for Health and Care Excellence (NICE) in relation to pregnant prisoners. However, NICE guidance does refer to female prisoners in broader guidance relating to smoking cessation, substance misuse, alcohol addiction and complex social needs [24, 25]. The importance of access to specially trained midwives for women with complex social needs is recommended (ibid). Women who are pregnant in prison, although in receipt of healthcare, have little or no choice over place of birth, birth partner or whether the baby remains with her [26–28]. Women are not told the date or times of hospital appointments (e.g. she will not be told the date of her scan for security purposes and will be accompanied by Prison Officers rather than a partner or family member) [4]. Due to the limited number of female prisons, it is likely that a woman will give birth far away from her home in an unfamiliar hospital [29]. She may have some provisions for labour, but these will be vetted by the prison

---

⁵Article 3 of the Human Rights Act states: 'you must not be tortured or treated in an inhuman or degrading way. Inhuman treatment is ill-treatment which causes you severe mental or physical suffering. The ill-treatment does not have to be deliberate or inflicted on purpose. Degrading treatment is treatment which is grossly humiliating or undignified' (Citizens Advice Bureau, 2017).

⁶A Prison Service Order (PSO) or Prison Service Instruction (PSI) is guidance as to how prison services are regulated.

service prior to transfer. Recent media interest [30] galvanised by the charity Birth Companions and the research of Abbott [31] has led to calls for policy change and making guidance for the care of perinatal women in prison mandatory.

8.5   Impact of Prison upon Health Behaviours

The impact on the health needs and health behaviour of the childbearing population in prison is multifaceted, and the complexities of the promotion of health for this group of women is challenging due to their vulnerabilities and potential lack of self-efficacy. The setting of the prison estate means that women are deprived of a basic level of control and could have reduced self-esteem thus reducing the chance of behaviour change. Being in prison and having a loss of control may also lead to a crisis point and therefore impact upon stress levels and make keeping mentally well a struggle. Seigman and Maier (1967) suggest that people who are threatened with a loss of control will try and regain it and, if they cannot, may exhibit "learned helplessness" and psychological dysfunction [32]. The woman in prisons' average demographic is someone who may be abusing substances, may have been in care, may have mental health problems and may have a poor diet, and therefore, health promotion may not have featured strongly within her life. Conversely, the prison setting may be the first time a woman with these characteristics has had a safe place to shelter, has organised mealtimes and bedtimes and has had access to healthcare and better nutrition. Therefore, it could be argued that self-efficacy may be increased for some and also may affect motivation for a change in behaviour [33]. Encouraging health behaviour changes such as stopping smoking and improving diet within the prison environment could be especially difficult due to lack of choice over food and ready accessibility of cigarettes, for example. Norman et al. (2005) [33] claim that the perception of the (woman's) own vulnerabilities will influence self-efficacy effecting motivation when attempting to change health behaviours.

8.6   Midwifery Care in Prison

Midwives, usually based in local community teams, provide antenatal care in the prison, monitoring the pregnancy and wellbeing of the woman, and visit women post birth, providing post-natal care [34]. Scans and specialist referrals are usually facilitated in the local hospital, and the woman will not be told the dates of appointments for security reasons. Women are usually accompanied by two prison officers unless she has been given permission for a hospital visit released on temporary license. When a woman's labour begins in prison, she will be transferred to the local hospital, usually accompanied by prison officers in a taxi or prison van. Following birth, depending on whether a woman has been awarded a place on an MBU, she will return either to a prison MBU with her baby or to the general prison without her baby.

8.7 Health Outcomes of Pregnant Women in Prison

When compared with a healthy non-prison population of women, imprisoned women have poorer outcomes. Nevertheless, when compared to similar disadvantaged groups of women, not in prison, physical outcomes for the babies such as birth weight and risk of stillbirth were improved, although the babies of women in prison were more likely to be born prematurely. In 2005, Knight and Plugge [35] compared the health outcomes of pregnant prisoners and their babies, to a similar group of women with complex needs, and who were not in prison. The findings suggested that having access to healthcare, accommodation and regular meals may have been the reason for improved outcomes. Bard et al. (2016) [36] reviewed the evidence with outcome-based evaluations, and the evaluations were outcome based, concluding that there were several missed opportunities to improve the health of pregnant women whilst they were incarcerated.

Following the Marmot Review, "Fair Society Healthy Lives", which considered health inequalities, with special consideration for the socially disadvantaged [37], Albertson et al. (2012) [26] initiated a consultation with healthcare and prison staff to elicit the views on pregnancy provisions, MBU experience and partnership working. The findings included inconsistency in care provision and communication breakdowns. Similar to previous reviews, it was reported that routine data was not collected, including accurate numbers of pregnant women in prison. Albertson et al. (2012) found that the prison system often negated information sharing and collaborative working due to issues around data protection, with the prison not wishing to share information about prisoners. Albertson et al. (2012) highlighted good practices that enhanced the service provision for pregnant women and new mothers, especially through charitable organisations.

8.8 Retrospective Health Outcomes for Pregnant Women in Prison

An exploration of retrospective data of incarcerated pregnant women and new mothers in Australia offered further insight into the health outcomes and demographics. A retrospective cohort study entitled "Mothers and gestation in custody" (MAGIC) explored the perinatal outcomes for incarcerated women in New South Wales, Australia [38]. The records of 558 pregnant prisoners over a period of 6 years were accessed in order to study the consequence of imprisonment on pregnancy outcomes for mother and baby. Records were reviewed of women who had been incarcerated for at least 5 days, linking to mental health disorders and drug and alcohol addiction. The study findings contradicted the conclusions of previous systematic reviews in that there was no connection found between incarceration improving perinatal outcomes. Equally, Walker et al. (2014) found that imprisoned women and babies were more likely to have poor health outcomes, including a greater risk of a baby being admitted to neonatal intensive care for

5 days or more and babies being of low birth weight. One conclusion is that the prison service is not adequately prepared to provide appropriate healthcare for a perinatal woman.

8.9 Intervention Programmes for Pregnant Women in Prison

Shroeder and Bell (2005) [39] developed an intervention programme whereby pregnant women in prison were assigned a doula[7] for labour and found where this kind of service is offered to incarcerated pregnant women elevated levels of satisfaction are recorded. The prison staff saw the service as "supportive" as they were able to proceed with their security role and felt less out of their depth when faced with the requirements of the pregnant inmate. Women reported their satisfaction of the additional support in labour. Themes from the interviews with women included the anticipation of loss following separation from their babies, hopes for the future and satisfaction of the support given by the doulas.

8.10 Qualitative Research into Pregnant Women's Experience of Prison

Four qualitative studies from the USA, eliciting pregnant women's experiences of incarceration, were discovered through literature searches. Research aims of all US studies followed a similar pattern and exposed themes within the maternal relationship with their unborn baby [40–42]. One UK qualitative study undertaken by Gardiner et al. (2016) [43] in Scotland sought the views of pregnant women and mothers in an MBU. No published studies analysing specifically the experience of pregnant women have been undertaken in the UK until Abbott's 2018 ethnographic study into the experiences of pregnant women in English prisons [44].

8.11 Connectedness with the Unborn Baby

Wismont's (2000) [45] study looked solely at women separated from their babies following birth through interviews with 12 women. Wismont encouraged women to use journals to record their thoughts and followed up with semi-structured interviews. The study uncovers themes of grief and loss but also a deep relationship with their unborn child: "connectedness". This connection was expressed despite the impending separation from the baby. The small sample offered a unique, in-depth examination of an aspect of pregnancy in prison and is one of the few qualitative

---

[7]A doula is a woman who provides support and gives advice to pregnant, birthing and post-natal women. Doulas are usually mothers themselves but have no professional qualification in midwifery.

studies of its kind. Of note was the women's sense of feeling valued and being able to keep the diaries which may have enhanced their feelings of self-worth when suffering the pain of loss.

8.12 Loss and Grief

Chambers (2009) [41] undertook interviews in an American prison looking specifically at attachment for women who would be forcibly separated from their babies at birth. Findings from data analysis from 12 participants developed into 4 main themes including "a love connection"; "everything was great until I birthed"; "feeling empty and missing part of me"; and "I don't try and think too far in advance". Like Wismont's findings, the theme of connectedness was strong, and of note, the threat to that "connectedness" came with the birth of the baby, whereas in the non-prison birthing encounter, bonding is increased at birth. Loss, grief and the inability to let go or face impending separation were articulated emotions. Interestingly, another finding exposed the staff/prisoner relationship; where the relationships were more positive with prison staff, the experience of separation from the baby was deemed to be less stressful.

8.13 Psychological Findings

Hutchinson et al.'s (2008) [46] research took a phenomenological approach comprising semi-structured audiotaped interviews and self-reporting questionnaires with 25 women. Twenty-one women were pregnant at the time of the interview, and four had given birth in prison a few months earlier. The interviews were held in one large room and conducted by four interviewers and included open-ended questions and administration of psychological tests. These methods included tests which measure maternal/baby bonding, psychological distress and the Beck Depression Inventory [47]. Findings included the fear of separation from the baby at birth, increased feelings of hostility in pregnancy and interpretation placing prison as an opportunity to elicit changing behaviours when pregnant. Loneliness, stress and depressive symptoms were consistent findings with all the women, suggesting that pregnant women in prison have specific difficulties that need enhanced support.

8.14 Separation Trauma

A Scottish qualitative study entitled "The Rose Project" pursued the views of staff and women about the experience of pregnancy and becoming a mother in prison [43], which concur with the assertions of Albertson et al. (2012) and O'Keefe and Dixon (2015) by sourcing the views of a variety of professionals. The trauma of separation from the baby was a consistent theme described by staff and women. The recommendations were like those of previous studies: the opportunity to use the experience of incarceration as a catalyst for change, additional and tailored support from professionals, alternatives to custody for pregnant women and mothers as well as further research with the wider family members such as fathers and grandparents.

8.15   Understanding the Experiences of Pregnant Women in Prison

Most of the previous studies recommend that perceptions of women be sought, yet the larger-scale research tended to focus on staff opinion. The qualitative studies that have gathered women's perceptions focus on the connection with the unborn baby and reflections of the pregnancy experience post release. The gap in the evidence prompted the research question, "What is women's experience of pregnancy in prison?", the aim being to capture subjective accounts leading to an understanding of women's own experiences of their pregnancy whilst incarcerated and from their perspective.

> **Lived Experience Perspective**
> "If I didn't have a birth companion it would have been horrible because you can't say to the midwife you can you rub my back for me they are in uniform but they are doing their job aren't they, so you need to see someone, it's nice to see someone just in plain clothes, you don't realise how much plain clothes mean."
> (Karima)

8.16   The Incarcerated Pregnancy

Abbott's ethnographic study took place over ten months during 2015–2016 and involved semi-structured interviews with 28 female prisoners in England who were pregnant or had recently given birth whilst imprisoned, 10 members of staff and a period of non-participant observation. Follow-up interviews with five women were undertaken as their pregnancies progressed to birth and the post-natal phase.

The findings suggest that pregnancy is an anomaly within the patriarchal prison system [31]. The main findings of the study are divided into four broad concepts, namely, (a) "institutional thoughtlessness" [48], whereby prison life continues with little thought for those with unique physical needs such as pregnant women, and (b) "institutional ignominy" [31] where the women experience "shaming" as a result of institutional practices which entail being displayed in public and adorned with institutional symbols of imprisonment. The study also revealed new information about the (c) coping strategies adopted by pregnant prisoners and (d) elucidated how the women navigate the system to negotiate entitlements and seek information about their rights [31].

> **Empathic Considerations**
> Close your eyes. Imagine your perspective of what a prison looks like and how it might feel to be inside. Envisage the environment and what the atmosphere may feel like. Now imagine a pregnant woman in her last trimester. Place her in that environment. Consider how she may be feeling. What do you think her worries and concerns may be?

8.17   Findings of My Research

The findings of my research led to considerations about the healthcare of the perinatal woman in prison. Women often discover their pregnancy on entry to prison; however, women report that they are unaware of their choices and options, especially if this is their first time in prison. Pregnancy symptoms can be especially difficult to manage. In my research, women described the discomforts of early pregnancy, especially in relation to food and nutrition, feeling nauseous and intense tiredness. Although women were not visibly pregnant, they often felt anxious about their unborn baby, having heard stories of miscarriage with feelings of disempowerment and fear of the unknown. Discrepancies were revealed regarding women gaining entitlements (e.g. proper nutrition and basic necessities such as breast pads). Women experienced shame and struggled with navigating prison bureaucracy.

First trimester needs include extreme tiredness, nausea, information options, entry shock, drugs and alcohol withdrawal (see Mill's Chap. 4 on substance abuse for further depth on drugs and alcohol).

> *I can't get any fresh air … I don't like it, because it's a smoking wing and I don't like the smell of smoke. it makes me feel sick.* (Lien)

In the *second trimester*, women often report feeling more physically healthy and less tired. This is the phase where women are often described as "blooming". However, for the pregnant woman in prison, her pregnancy becomes visible to other prisoners, and this can make her feel vulnerable.

> *I try to hide my bump … I feel worried in case someone tries to hurt my baby, so I wear loose clothes … there are girls that are going in and out in and out and they want to touch your bump and you know you can't say to them "can you not do that please" cos it's like you don't know what they are in for.* (Tamsin)

> **Question to Consider**
> Why might a pregnant woman in prison be concerned about her pregnancy becoming more visible?

The woman entering the *third trimester* is preparing for labour and birth. In my research, I found that most women received information from prison staff and other inmates and did not have access to the information that many women may do due to Internet and social media [44, 49]. Women would describe how they felt scared about going into labour, especially at night-time. Stories would often spread quickly around the prisons about women not getting to hospital on time. Although women were entitled to have a birth partner with them in labour, due to the geographical locations of the prison in relation to family members, this was often not possible, also causing anxiety. Where women have the support from organisations such as Birth Companions (see Chaps. 2, 12 and 13 by Delap, Marshall and Ayers on how charitable organisations support women in prison) who provide women in prison with a birthing partner, this can make all the difference.

> "I just had enough being on the streets … when I went to prison it was the first time, I'd had my own bed, I finally got a routine back. I used to love the antenatal groups with Birth Companions … for the time I was with them, I felt like a normal pregnant woman, just for a few hours … Having the support from X during labour meant I was not on my own … I felt cared for and that my choices were listened to … I did not feel like just another prisoner, it made all the difference." (Karis, a woman supported by the charity Birth Companions)

> **Compassion in Action**
> "It's not until you look back and see, the little groups … they were so important in there, just being able to talk to someone, just something little, you know, just like I have never had a baby before, how will I know I am in labour? … so it means a lot, that somebody actually cares—'cos there are people like, I was, which was totally alone."
> (Frances)

8.18 Labour and Birth Options

In the ethnographic research, most women did not have access to pregnancy groups and got most of their information about choices from other women [44]. The majority had given birth before, and many women told me that they were anxious about having a precipitous (fast) birth.

> "I'm anxious about labour, because I know people that have died in labour. Not just that, I'm just scared of going in labour in here. I'd rather just get booked in and so I can just quickly have a caesarean". (Frida)

"I am a bit worried about what is going to happen. What's going to happen, I don't know, am I going to go intto labour on my own, am I going to be left in my cell, who will I get with me?" (Aiko)

Where women gave birth vaginally in hospital, they were often accompanied by prison officers which could be a comfort to some women, especially if a female officer they knew and trusted. Often women would choose a specific officer, and there were officers who liked to go on "bed watch" [50] with women.

8.19 Post-Natal Period

50% of women giving birth whilst incarcerated will be able to remain with their babies in one of the six MBUs in the UK. Women usually return to work or education at 6 weeks post-natal, and there are currently no official guidelines for maternity leave [5, 31]. Women on MBUs can bond with their babies, and the MBU is often within the main prison but away from the prison general population. Babies are not prisoners and are therefore able to be taken out of the prison to visit relatives or attend groups with nursery workers. Specially trained staff are usually on the MBUs, and women report a variety of positive and negative experiences. Family days enable siblings and partners to attend. However, the MBU environment albeit more pleasant to the rest of the main prison can be a place of tension. Women would tell me that they often felt like a "coiled spring" unable to release their true feelings for fear of reproaches:

"part of you wants to blow up but you can't because if you blow up you because something will happen, your baby gets taken from you, you know there is always a consequence to everything … you know everything you say, there is a consequence whether it is good or bad".

8.20 Separation

The other 50% of women will have their babies removed shortly after birth, often within 48 h. Some women chose to express breast milk for their unborn babies [27]. The complex emotions experienced, meant that a quick return to prison was sometimes chosen by women in order to blend back into the general prison population. Women would describe their despair and anguish and how they missed their baby. Expressing breast milk was a way of maintaining a bond, feeling useful and like a mother (ibid).

I got to spend two days with him, but when the midwives held him, and the officers held him he just cried. He only stopped crying when I had him…it was just the worst thing watching him being taken away and I haven't seen him since. (Janet)

8.21   Professional Considerations

When considering the perinatal woman in prison, it may be a useful exercise in our own unconscious bias to contemplate the following scenarios:

> You are sitting in a hospital waiting room with your young niece. A woman walks in wearing a grey baggy tracksuit, visibly pregnant accompanied by two prison officers. They sit opposite you.

> You are attending an antenatal appointment at 30 weeks gestation. You are an inmate in HMP Clifton serving a 12-month sentence for assisting an offender (your boyfriend) and accompanied by two prison officers who have just removed your handcuffs. The woman opposite you has a young child with her who she holds tightly averting her eyes from yours. Others are looking at you quizzically, nobody smiles. You feel very embarrassed and ashamed and try not to cry.

8.22   Conclusions

Women in prison are often survivors of childhood abuse, may have been in the care of the local authority, experienced homelessness and domestic abuse and misused drugs and alcohol. It is understood that as many as 80% of women in prison are diagnosed with mental ill health. It is understood that the numbers of pregnant women in prison are not collected, yet they are a group who may have considerable health needs due to often coming from a background of extreme disadvantage. This chapter has explored the evidence from current research exposing the health impacts and outcomes for pregnant prisoners and their babies. Qualitative research has uncovered the experiences of women in relation to human rights, connectedness with their unborn baby, the potential for toxic stress and underlying experiences of shame. The chapter considered experiences of the woman through vignettes, and the reader was asked to consider pre-conceived notions and examine potential bias. Recommendations for professional practice have been made.

References

1. Walmsley R. World prison population list. World prison brief. Birkbeck: Institute for Criminal Policy Research, International Centre for Prison Studies, University of London; 2013.
2. Gerry F, Harris L. Women in prison: is the justice system fit for purpose? Halsbury Law Exchange; 2016. http://blogs.lexisnexis.co.uk/halsburyslawexchange/wp-content/uploads/sites/25/2016/11/SA-1016-077-Women-in-Prison-Paper-ONLINE-FINAL.pdf

3. Albertson K, O'Keefe C, Burke C, Lessing-Turner G Renfrew M. Addressing health inequalities for mothers and babies in prison. Health and inequality: applying public health research to policy and practice; 2014, p. 39

4. Abbott L. A pregnant pause: expecting in the prison estate. In: Baldwin L, editor. Mothering justice: working with mothers in criminal and social justice settings. 1st ed. England: Waterside Press; 2015.

5. Kennedy A, Marshall D, Parkinson D, Delap N, Abbott L. Birth charter for women in prison in England and Wales. London: Birth Companions; 2016.

6. Prison Reform Trust. Bromley briefings, prison: the facts. London: Prison Reform Trust; 2018.   http://www.prisonreformtrust.org.uk/Portals/0/Documents/Bromley%20Briefings/ Summer%202018%20factfile.pdf

7. Abbott L. Pregnant female offenders behind bars. In: Frailing K, editor. Encyclopedia of women and crime. Wiley-Blackwell; 2019. https://doi.org/10.1002/9781118929803. ewac0412

8. Ministry of Justice. Population and capacity briefing. London: Ministry of Justice; 2019.

9. North J, Chase L, Alliance M. Getting it right: services for pregnant women, new mothers, and babies in prison: Lankelly Chase; 2006.

10. Corston J. The Corston report: a report by Baroness Jean Corston of a review of women with particular vulnerabilities in the criminal justice system: the need for a distinct, radically different, visibly-led, strategic, proportionate, holistic, woman-centred, integrated approach. Home Office; 2007.

11. Baldwin L, O'Malley S, Galway K. Mothers addicted: working with complexity. Chapter 10. In: Baldwin L, editor. Mothering justice: working with mothers in social and criminal justice settings; 2015, pp. 239–262.

12. Baldwin L, Epstein R. Short but not sweet: a study of the imposition of short custodial sentences on women, and in particular, on mothers. De Montfort University; 2017.

13. Gullberg S. State of the estate—women in prison's report on the women's custodial estate 2011-12. London: Women in Prison; 2013.

14. United Nations. The Bangkok rules; 2013. http://www.penalreform.org/priorities/women-in-the-criminal-justice-system/bangkok-rules-2/

15. Council of Europe. Committee of Ministers. European Prison Rules. Council of Europe. Recommendation Rec. 2 of the Committee of Ministers to member states on the European Prison Rules; 2006.

16. UN General Assembly. The universal declaration of human rights. Resolution adopted by the General Assembly 10/12. New York: United Nations; 1948.

17. Schiller R. Why human rights in childbirth matter. Pinter and Martin; 2016.

18. Plimmer G. Care UK becomes biggest prison health care provider. Financial Times; 9th May 2016.

19. Parveen N. Prisons ombudsman investigates death of new mother taken off suicide watch. The Guardian; 2016. https://www.theguardian.com/society/2016/feb/09/new-mother-killed-herself-prison-shortly-after-taken-off-suicide-watch?CMP=share_btn_gp

20. Abbott L, Delap N. Holding the baby: responsibility for addressing the needs of offending pregnant women and new mothers should be shared across the system. Howard League Penal Reform Early Career Acad Netw Bull. 2016;31:34–40.

21. Bosely S. The Guardian (International), United Kingdom, Print. https://www.theguardian. com/society/2018/nov/13/female-prisoners-in-england-left-to-give-birth-alone-in-their-cells-report-reveals. Accessed 13 Nov 2018.

22. Devlin H, Taylor D. The Guardian (International), United Kingdom, Print. https://www.the-guardian.com/society/2019/oct/04/baby-dies-in-uk-prison-after-inmate-gives-birth-alone-in-cell. Accessed 04 Oct 2019.

23. Royal College of Midwives. Caring for childbearing prisoners: a position paper. Position statement for women in custody. London; 2016.

24. National Institute for Health and Clinical Excellence (NICE). Pregnancy and complex social factors: a model for service provision for pregnant women with complex social factors. NICE; 2010. http://www.nice.org.uk/guidance/cg110

25. National Institute for Health and Clinical Excellence (NICE). Pregnancy and complex social factors overview. NICE; 2014. http://pathways.nice.org.uk/pathways/pregnancy-and-complexsocialfactors

26. Albertson, K., O'Keefe, C., Lessing-Turner, G., Burke, C., Renfrew, M. J. Tackling health inequalities through developing evidence-based policy and practice with childbearing women in prison: a consultation. The Hallam Centre for Community Justice, Sheffield Hallam University and The Mother and Infant Research Unit, University of York; 2012.

27. Abbott L, Scott T. Women's experiences of breastfeeding in prison. MIDIRS Midwifery Digest. 2017;27(2):217–23.

28. Sikand M. Lost spaces: is the current provision for women prisoners to gain a place in a prison mother and baby unit fair and accessible? The Griffins Society University of Cambridge Institute of Criminology; 2017.

29. Galloway S, Haynes A, Cuthbert C. All babies count—an unfair sentence: spotlight on the criminal justice system. London: NSPCC; 2015.

30. https://www.theguardian.com/society/2018/nov/13/female-prisoners-in-england-left-to-give-birth-alone-in-their-cells-report-reveals

31. Abbott L, Scott T, Thomas H, Weston K. Pregnancy and childbirth in English prisons: institutional ignominy and the pains of imprisonment. Sociol Health Illness. 2020;42(3):660–75.

32. Seigman MEP, Maier SF. Failure to escape traumatic shock. J Exp Psychol. 1967;74:1–9.

33. Norman P; Boer H, Seydel ER. Protection motivation theory in Connor and Norman (2005) predicting health behaviour. 2nd ed. Open University Press; 2005.

34. Kennedy A, Marshall D, Parkinson D, Delap N, Abbott L. Birth charter for women in prisons in England and Wales. Birth Companions; 2016.

35. Knight M, Plugge E. The outcomes of pregnancy among imprisoned women: a systematic review. Br J Obstet Gynaecol. 2005;112(11):1467–74.

36. Bard E, Knight M, Plugge E. Perinatal health care services for imprisoned pregnant women and associated outcomes: a systematic review. BMC Pregnancy Childbirth. 2016;16(1):285.

37. Marmot MG. Fair society, healthy lives: the marmot review. Executive summary: strategic review of health inequalities in England Post-2010; 2010.

38. Walker JR, Hilder L, Levy MH, Sullivan EA. Pregnancy, prison and perinatal outcomes in New South Wales, Australia: a retrospective cohort study using linked health data. BMC Pregnancy Childbirth. 2014;14(1):1.

39. Schroeder C, Bell J. Doula birth support for incarcerated pregnant women. Public Health Nurs. 2005;22(1):53–8.

40. Wismont JM. The lived pregnancy experience of women in prison. J Midwifery Womens Health. 2000;45(4):292–300.

41. Chambers AN. Impact of forced separation policy on incarcerated postpartum mothers. Policy Politics Nurs Pract. 2009;10(3):204–11.

42. Fritz S, Whiteacre K. Prison nurseries: experiences of incarcerated women during pregnancy. J Offender Rehabilit. 2016;55(1):1–20.

43. Gardiner A, Daniel B, Burgess C, Nolan L. The rose project: best for babies-determining and supporting the best interests and wellbeing of babies of imprisoned mothers in Scotland. University of Stirling; 2016.

44. Abbott LJ. The incarcerated pregnancy: an ethnographic study of perinatal women in English prisons. University of Hertfordshire; 2018.

45. Wismont JM. The lived pregnancy experience of women in prison. J Midwifery and Women's Health. 2000;45(4):292–300.

46. Hutchinson KC, Moore GA, Propper CB, Mariaskin A. Incarcerated women's psychological functioning during pregnancy. Psychol Women Quart. 2008;32(4):440–53.

47. Beck AT, Steer RA, Brown G. Beck depression inventory–II. Psychological assessment. Jan 1, 1996.
48. Crawley E. Institutional thoughtlessness in prisons and its impacts on the day-to-day prison lives of elderly men. J Contemp Criminal Justice. 2005;21(4):350–63.
49. Borrelli SE, Walsh D, Spiby H. First-time mothers' choice of birthplace: influencing factors, expectations of the midwife's role and perceived safety. J Adv Nurs. 2017;73:1937–46.
50. Abbott L. Escorting pregnant prisoners-the experiences of women and staff. Prison Serv J. 2019;241:20.

Pregnant Refugees and Asylum Seekers

9

Carolyn Hill

Abstract

This chapter will offer some insight to the range of issues faced by pregnant women as they seek asylum and refuge in the UK. Migration poses several challenges related to the care and treatment of pregnant women and their access to services. The rise in conflict both within and between nation states and global warming, resulting in natural disasters and financial depression, have all led to an increased global displacement of people numbering close to 70 million. Of this number, 25.4 million are refugees, and 3.1 million are asylum seekers, comprising of individuals and small communities fleeing persecution on the grounds of race, religion, political or other beliefs and practices in search of sanctuary in other countries. Just under half of this number is women. Data from the office of the United Nations High Commissioner for Refugees (UNHCR; https://www.unhcr.org/uk/figures-at-a-glance.html) indicated 57% of refugees come from three countries: Afghanistan, South Sudan and Syria (UNHCR; https://www.unhcr.org/uk/figures-at-a-glance.html), currently placing the flight from conflict as the highest factor for displacement. Within the UK, the number of asylum seekers has seen a reduction on previous years' applications. By June 2018, the UK Home Office (UK Home Office; https://www.gov.uk/government/publications/immigration-statistics-year-ending-june-2018/how-many-people-do-we--grant-asylum-or-protection-to#key-facts) had issued just over 14,000 grants of asylum. The processes of migration and seeking refuge impact the wellbeing of this already vulnerable group of women increasing inequalities in health and social outcomes for them and their children.

C. Hill (✉)
Division of Social Work Community and Public Health, Institute of Health and Social Care, London South Bank University, London, UK
e-mail: hillc13@lsbu.ac.uk

© Springer Nature Switzerland AG 2021
L. Abbott (ed.), *Complex Social Issues and the Perinatal Woman*,
https://doi.org/10.1007/978-3-030-58085-8_9

Keywords

Asylum seeker · Refugee · Migration · Housing · Access to maternity care

This chapter outlines and hopefully increases some awareness in the reader of some of the many issues that the perinatal woman, seeking refuge, may encounter. It begins with the process of seeking asylum and the difficulties associated with providing evidence of being an asylum seeker. There is a brief focus on housing, benefits and access to healthcare, highlighting the misconceptions held by many in the host country that asylum seekers and refugees jump to the head of the housing queue, receive better financial support than others already living in the UK and are only in the country to make use of our beloved National Health Service. Matters focusing around the violence some women may have suffered and their physical health are discussed alongside issues of psychological trauma. It stops short of discussing the importance of trauma-informed care, as this is addressed elsewhere in this book. However, the same principles of providing care holistically, sensitive to the needs of each individual woman in a compassionate, non-judgemental manner through a concerted collaboration with other health- and social care professionals and voluntary organisation, remain highly applicable.

9.1   Definitions

Asylum seeker: 'A fundamental human right, under international law is the right to seek asylum, in any country, as set out in article 14(1)' [1]. *The Universal Declaration on Human Rights remains unequivocal in this matter.* So, what is an asylum seeker? In the UK, an asylum seeker is someone who has made an application to the government to obtain refugee status; while they are awaiting the decision, they are considered as asylum seekers, in a state of 'sanctuary' away from their country of origin. At the end of 2017, there were approximately 40,000 asylum seekers in the UK. The granting of asylum and refugee status can be a prolonged and complex process. The Home Office has the right to grant asylum. However, not all claims for asylum are granted, and in 2017, up to 41% of the claims for asylum, which were initially rejected by the Home Office, were eventually overturned by the appeals courts. This overturning follows very stringent appeals procedures [2, 3], during which there remains an uncertainty of asylum status. This type of delay adds to the stresses already encountered by this vulnerable group of people.

   Refugee: In the UK, once an asylum seeker has their claim for asylum granted by the Home Office, they are acknowledged as a refugee and have the incumbent rights. This means that under the principle of 'non-refoulment' they will not be sent back to the country from which they fled. The universal definition assigned by the 1951 Refugee Convention was couched in legal terms but is offered here as *someone who is unable or unwilling to return to their country of origin owing to a* *well-founded fear of being persecuted for reasons of race, religion, nationality, membership of a particular social group, or political opinion*[1]. One can begin to see where and how some confusion arises between the terms 'asylum seeker' and 'refugee'. Once granted refugee status, they have the right to seek employment and claim benefits. For refugees with families who remained in the country of origin, it also means that their children (under the age of 18 years) and partners may join them in the UK.

This may be a step in the right direction to what may be a more stable life but is initially fraught with challenges. As refugees, they now need to give up (within 21 days) the temporary accommodation they were housed in as asylum seekers, and their subsistence allowance ceases by the end of that time too. It means that they run the risk of becoming homeless until they can find a suitable place to reside. Subsequently, until they have an address, they cannot apply for jobs, open bank accounts or claim benefits. However, support is available from local councils and charities with the provision of emergency accommodation, until more permanent accommodation can be secured.

Migrant: Asylum seekers and refuges may be considered as migrants under the definition offered by the IOM: 'any person who is moving or has moved across an international border or within a State away from his/her habitual place of residence, regardless of (1) the person's legal status; (2) whether the movement is voluntary or involuntary; (3) what the causes for the movement are; or (4) what the length of the stay is'[4]. The terms have been used interchangeably by the media and governments alike, and as yet, there is no internationally accepted legal definition of a migrant [5], so it is important to make some distinction between them. However, it is more generally accepted that migrants move to countries to find employment rather than flee from perilous situations within their home countries, and as such, migrants are likely to be of working age, generally more educated and in good health [6].

9.2   The Process of Seeking Asylum in the UK [7]

On arrival in the UK, the asylum seeker must notify the border force officer that they are seeking asylum and their reasons for doing so. This usually occurs at the point of entry to the country. The reasons for seeking asylum must fulfil the eligibility criteria (fear of persecution, breach of human rights) for their claim to be considered. Documents such as a passport and other forms of identification (marriage certificate, police registration certificates) need to be provided to instigate an initial screening interview with an immigration officer. This poses many problems, especially if the woman has fled with few of any personal possessions; if these documents are not available, the process is delayed at this point until the border force agency is able to verify the authenticity for seeking asylum. At the screening interview, following preliminary checks about possible previous applications for asylum to other countries, the claimant is given an application reference number. At this initial screening interview, a woman will be asked specifically if she may be pregnant, and her reasons for seeking asylum are also discussed. Following the screening meeting, a case worker is appointed and an 'asylum registration card' issued. The asylum registration card may be used as a form of identification and importantly entitles access to education and healthcare.

The case worker is responsible for making a decision about the asylum application. The time taken to make a decision can take up to 6 months, more often much longer, and 'leave to remain' may be granted under one of two categories: as a refugee or on humanitarian grounds for protection. Both categories entitle the recipient to settle in the UK after a period of 5 years. If the initial application for asylum is rejected, the applicants have a right to appeal, and legal aid is available although limited.

9.3   Housing and Accommodation

Whilst their claim for asylum is being considered, they are entirely reliant on the government's support. This 'asylum support' takes the form of housing, with no choice as to where they may live, with many living in 'shared accommodation' alongside a mix of other asylum seekers. The housing and accommodation system falls under the jurisdiction of the Home Office and is subcontracted to companies such as G4S and Serco for housing provision [8]. Asylum seekers may initially be housed in hostels and hotels or reception centres, providing free 'full board' facilities, if a suitable space is available [9]. The use of detention centres has been restricted, but these are still in use when there is no other suitable accommodation immediately available. In a 2013 report by Feldman [10], women describe these detention centres as 'prisons', with atmospheres related to intimidation and fear. The criteria for using a detention centre are specific and include aspects related to the risk of an asylum seeker absconding and being 'lost' to the system whilst awaiting the Home Office decision.

Asylum seekers may be placed in 'initial accommodation', which has limited capacity, until more suitable 'dispersal accommodation' can be found in specific designated areas of the UK. Consideration of the individual's health needs is made, and a referral is made to the Initial Accommodation Healthcare Team when a 'treating clinician' or other appropriate healthcare professionals (midwife/health visitor) are notified as soon as possible of the woman's arrival. At this point, the midwife/nurse will offer health screening to include for infectious/communicable conditions such as TB, HIV and hepatitis A, B and C. If a woman is accompanied by her children, they too are screened, and their immunisation status is determined. Following a recording of maternity history, a pregnancy test will be carried out to confirm pregnancy and sexual health issues elicited for further treatment or advice.

It is the case worker's responsibility to ensure all information relating to the individual's health status and needs are clearly documented and reported to the relevant agency to maintain some continuity of care. This becomes especially important as the 'dispersal' accommodation is not in the same location as the 'initial' (emergency/temporary) accommodation, as it may mean registering with a different

GP and for maternity services in the new area. The 'dispersal accommodation providers' are required (by the Home Office) to assist the woman, with registering with a local GP and with information related to other health services (appointments maternity care). The case worker may also liaise with the local authority services to provide additional help in the form of social care.

For those pregnant women who disclose or screen positive for communicable conditions, dispersal to an area with appropriate healthcare provision is made to ensure that once care and treatment are initiated, they may continue in the same area to minimise further risk to the woman, but also to manage the condition from a public health perspective of preventing further transmission (e.g. mother to baby transmission; services already available for managing children with HIV) and supporting those with the condition to adhere to treatment.

The dispersal of pregnant women should be kept to an absolute minimum. However, Feldman [10] reported that many women were still be moved within the UK Border Agency's restricted period of 36 weeks gestation to four weeks postpartum. The instability created by multiple moves through the dispersal process, at a time when a woman feels at her most vulnerable, gives rise to isolation. The woman's ability to develop friendship and support networks with others in a similar situation is diminished, as she is separated from any networks she may have established. This has the potential to deepen any underlying psychological trauma. The morbidities from other underlying health issues can be exacerbated, as the access to health services in a new area is negotiated again and new appointments made. Some women in Feldman's study [10] reported giving birth alone, without a birth partner or interpreter present.

9.4   Financial Support and Benefits

As a rule, asylum seekers are not entitled to work. The Immigration and Asylum Act 1999 enables financial support. The National Asylum Support Service [11] entitles asylum seekers to claim some financial support which currently amounts to just over £5 a day (£37.75 per week) for general subsistence, e.g. food and clothing [12]. The application for this consists of a 35-page form in English and enquires about assets that may be liquidated to provide immediate funds. In many ways, this seems to be quite an insensitive enquiry, as many may have fled their home countries with very few material possessions. However, applicants have to prove that they are destitute in order to receive the subsistence allowance. In exceptional circumstances, where their application has been pending a decision for more than a year, special permission may be sought form the Home Office to apply for jobs from a restricted list [13].

Pregnant asylum seekers and refugees may apply to receive 'Asylum Support' and a one-off 'maternity payment' of £300 per baby [13]. Until they have been granted leave to remain, no other benefits may be claimed. This leaves many women exposed to poverty and destitution and vulnerable to exploitation. Some support in the provision of 'essentials' may be sought from and offered by local charities.

9.5   Access to Healthcare

Access to healthcare services for asylum seekers and refugees remains a contentious issue [14] due to society's perceptions, fuelled by media reports, of migrants wanting to take advantage of the British healthcare system. Only a very small number of asylum seekers are aware of the provision of healthcare through the NHS [15]. Some asylum seekers and refugees have been refused the opportunity of registering with a GP as they were not able to provide the relevant documents (asylum registration card), which enables access to the NHS. However, they are freely entitled to the following healthcare services:

• Registering with a GP, including secondary care for urgent treatment
• Accident and emergency care
• Antenatal care
• Mental health care and treatment under the Mental Health Act 1983
• Secondary care for urgent treatment
• Sexual health and family planning services
• Treatment for communicable conditions (TB, malaria, HIV/AIDS)

The study by Oliver [16] relating predominantly to migrant workers demonstrated a general lack of clarity for health- and social care service providers with regard to the entitlement of free healthcare. The UK Department of Health has guidance [17] on the availability of healthcare to asylum seekers and refugees; the guidance is slightly different in each UK nation, so it's worth checking the Department of Health website depending on where you may be practising. The Department of Health states health services for asylum seekers and refugees are free of charge; however, the Home office does place some restrictions with the exception of a very few cases [18] (as this site is updated, it is best to check who may not be exempted from charges for NHS care and treatment). Asylum seekers whose initial application for refugee status may have been rejected are still entitled to free healthcare and treatment, albeit for a very limited period. This access to free healthcare applies to maternity care [13].

The vast majority of problems identified by asylum seekers relate to issues of access to services, language barriers, relationships with health professionals and the acceptability of medical care, based on cultural beliefs and expectations [19].

The language barrier poses a significant problem when trying to access healthcare. This is not exclusively limited to verbal communication, when trying to make an appointment by telephone, but also to written materials and is especially problematic when forms need to be completed. Although the provision of interpreters has been longstanding in the NHS, their availability can be limited and inconsistent. Within some primary care settings, there has been some confusion about who is responsible for the organisation and payment of professional interpreting services [19]. This makes the provision of interpreting services inconsistent and patchy, leaving those seeking treatment dissatisfied and frustrated at not being able to fully explain their problems, consequently receiving inadequate care and treatment and further adding to their health burden. Women have also reported being concerned about the quality of interpreting services and the confidentiality that should be afforded to them [2]. They felt that interpreters were not representing their conditions accurately, potentially creating errors for misdiagnosis, as well as inadequate explanations of treatment or medical terms. Interpreters may be drawn from a similar community as that of the woman, and many women remain fearful of personal and confidential information being shared with members of their community.

Many asylum seekers and refugees feel discriminated against, making them fearful of seeking advice and treatment. These feelings arise from the attitudes that they experience in their interactions with health personnel, be it a receptionist or doctor, in person or on the telephone. They feel that their concerns are minimised and not understood and that there is a general lack of interest [19]. Women valued interactions with people who treated them holistically. Their preference was for health professionals who afforded them time to express themselves and their problems, were sympathetic to their plight and demonstrated some understanding of their cultural and religious beliefs and gender, treating them with respect and dignity. They appreciated the ability to see the same health professional as a means of building some rapport and trust to provide continuity of care.

When moved from their initial accommodation to dispersal accommodation, asylum seekers and refugees are supported by the initial accommodation healthcare team to register with a local GP to enable access to other health services. However, it is not only transport to and from hospital appointments that limits their attendance and access to treatment but also having to renegotiate some of the appointments for speciality services. Once at the hospital or maternity centre, signs can be confusing, and locating specific departments or rooms for the consultation may also create a sense of confusion and feeling 'lost'.

This leaves already vulnerable women in a precarious position, especially where pregnancy and maternity care are concerned. The lack of clarity is further compounded by issues of limited services around certain areas of residence ('post code lottery') and poor access as mentioned above, due to inadequate transportation; the inverse care law is still very much in evidence. These factors are further impeded by language barriers as well as the attitudes and beliefs held by some in the host population and by some health- and social care workers, related to asylum seekers and refugees 'abusing' the NHS and becoming a burden on the welfare system in their need to seek advice, treatment and care.

The National Institute for Health and Care Excellence [20] clearly recognised the complex issues facing pregnant, asylum-seeking women and their poor health outcomes. The guidance is clear in directing healthcare providers to ensure that any potential barriers such as language difficulties and understanding how to access maternity services are addressed using appropriate means (e.g. use of an interpreter or different communication methods, posters, videos), as well as identifying their own training needs to provide appropriate care and treatment. NICE [21] advocates a multi-agency approach to the care of a pregnant asylum seeker.

9.6   Physical Health

The Mothers and Babies: Reducing Risk through Audits and Confidential Enquiries across the UK (MBRRACE-UK) report (2018) [22] identified vulnerable groups of women, amongst whom asylum seekers and refugees are counted. These women suffer disproportionately higher rates of maternal and neonatal morbidity and mortality when compared to the host population. Prioritisation of the asylum-seeking process, alongside cultural and religious beliefs about health, pregnancy and childbirth, may offer some limited insight to the reasons for delayed seeking of antenatal care. More pertinent factors, for the delay and low engagement with maternity and health services, would be issues related to language barriers and poor availability of interpreting services, frequent moves to different dispersal accommodation areas and limited access to and understanding of UK health systems. Women who arrive in the host country in the later stages of their pregnancy are at greatest risk of poor pregnancy and birth outcomes [23].

Overall maternal and neonatal outcomes are reported to be poorer than the host population due to increased Caesarean sections, eclampsia, postpartum haemorrhage, low birth weight, pre-term deliveries, congenital anomalies and higher rates of admission to neonatal intensive care units. Pre-, peri- and post-asylum-seeking stressors all negatively impact perinatal mental health [24].

In relation to the general rates of morbidity and mortality experienced by 'migrants', the literature offers contrasting evidence. Aldridge et al. suggest [25] that 'mortality advantage' is experienced by some migrants indicating that causes of death were lower in migrants, with better life expectancy outcomes than the host country population. The same systematic review [25], despite assessing data from six European countries (including the UK), acknowledges the scarcity of data specific to asylum seekers, refugees and forced migrants but stated that refugees too have a mortality advantage over the host population. However, although the data demonstrated an advantage in refugees, asylum seekers have a distinct disadvantage, suffering higher rates of mortality than the host population. The possible reasons for this may be the stability that ensues once claims for asylum have been granted, but, to date, there is little if any evidence to support this.

Women may have had access to healthcare within their own countries, but given that some may come from marginalised communities and left their country of origin for reasons of persecution, their use of such services may have been limited. Women may present with a host of underlying health problems ranging from physical injuries; infections such as TB, hepatitis and HIV; and long-term conditions such as diabetes. The importance of a thorough and systematic assessment of health needs is crucial to ensure correct care and treatment are instigated to safeguard the woman's health and pregnancy. There is an acknowledgement within the literature [26] that traditional beliefs and cultural practices play a fundamental role in influencing the access to healthcare in the home country. These cultural beliefs are deeply held and may influence how some women perceive Western, medicalised approaches to pregnancy and childbirth. It is important to elicit and understand the individual woman's cultural beliefs and perceptions about health, pregnancy and childbirth

[27], so she may be informed about the Western biomedical approach and a balance be drawn to reduce possible fears about engaging with health services in the host country.

The initial meeting to assess health needs and any associated physical examinations and investigations run the risk of re-traumatising any woman who may have suffered previous violence or abuse, so a very careful and sensitive approach is required [28] to minimise the risks associated with post-traumatic stress disorder. If they have suffered any form of trauma, they may only want to engage with female staff [19]. Consistency of staff is especially valued by these vulnerable women; it reduces the need to repeat their stories, assists with reducing their fear and anxiety of health service processes and begins to engender a degree of trust and even a sense of empowerment [29] through developing a therapeutic relationship. Building trust may take more time than is available; nonetheless, it should be provided to ensure their health needs are assessed and met as best as possible.

It is vital to understand at what stage the pregnancy is and how the woman became pregnant in the first place: was it a planned pregnancy or the result of rape? The woman's choice to continue with the pregnancy will need to be discussed with great sensitivity, as in some cultures and religions, termination of pregnancy for any reason is forbidden. Similarly, in cases of modern slavery and where sexual exploitation may be an underlying factor, a careful approach to eliciting the nature of conception needs to be employed. Ideally, the woman should be interviewed in a private setting, away from anyone, including 'friends' and 'partners'/husbands accompanying her, to enable a frank and open discussion with the health professional. This presents problems as the stigma associated with sexual violence is also likely to hinder its disclosure, and many women need to feel they can trust someone before any disclosure of abuse or violence is made. Women who require interpreters already have suspicions about the quality and trustworthiness of the interpretation services [2]. However, none of the people accompanying the woman should be used as an interpreter as this has the potential to inhibit and prevent disclosure of potential abuses.

The separation from family and friends (due to fleeing the home country or because of their death) may be acutely felt when pregnant. This lack of support at a time when families, regardless of ethnicity, culture or religion, come together to acknowledge and celebrate a pregnancy can impact the woman's mental health and trigger feelings of isolation and heightened vulnerability. Conversely, if the pregnancy is because of sexual violence, the possibility of social stigmatisation and risk of rejection by the family group is high [30], increasing the likelihood of depression and suicide ideation. Viewing these vulnerable women's health holistically is important to begin to address the inequalities experienced by them especially around the perinatal period, when women tend to feel at their most vulnerable.

Provision of and access to culturally sensitive care from the point of first contact have been identified by NICE [20] as fundamental to improving health outcomes for this group of women. This is also reflected in the wider, more contemporary literature assessing the health needs of all asylum seekers and refugees, not just women [19, 28]. Developing an understanding of an individual's background and situation is a basic premise to providing person-centred care and maintaining and rebuilding what dignity they may have left. Working effectively across professional and informal boundaries to ensure continuity of care and support addresses not only the physical aspects of health but also the social and psychological factors that influence it. Novick [31] suggested an approach that enables the person to tell their story, rather than relying on assessment tools, templates and investigations to glean information. Interactions where people have been allowed to talk and been attentively listened to reduce feelings of inadequacy and increase involvement in their care, subsequently enhancing the development of trust and empowerment [32].

Interactions that focus solely on a biomedical approach to assessing and addressing the individual woman's health needs run the risk of belittling the situation and possibly not addressing any underlying causes for poor health [28], an example of which may be a trafficked woman presenting with sexually transmitted infections because she may have been or is still being exploited as a sex worker. A coordinated multi-agency approach is not only central but vital in the process of meeting the health needs from a holistic perspective.

9.7   Violence

Sexual (rape) and physical violence including torture have a long history in war as a means of subjugation, to demoralise and control whole sections of society or communities, with devastating physical and psychological effects on the victims [33, 34]. Asylum seekers and refugees have high rates of post-traumatic stress disorder and depression as a consequence of these life-threatening events [35]. In the home country, women may have suffered repeated rapes with the sequelae of pregnancies resulting in miscarriages, sexually transmitted infections [36] and some long-term gynaecological health problems, with the added encumbrance of future sexual dysfunction. In many cases of rape and sexual violence, the breast tissue (papillae) is damaged too, leading to necrosis and the inability to breastfeed [34].

En route to a host country, women reported further sexual violence and exploitation as a means of paying for their transport [8]. Unfortunately, for many female asylum seekers and refugees, the abuse does not end on arrival in the host country. Some continue to suffer abuse/intimate partner violence in the host country. Baillot and Connelly [8] found that whilst under the asylum support system in the UK (i.e. awaiting refugee status), some of their claims of abuse and violence were not treated as 'serious' by case workers, who were reluctant to believe women's stories. Where some support was available (place of safety), it was fragile and inconsistent, based on limited availability of safe housing and accommodation in specific dispersal areas, which left women still vulnerable to access by their abuser even once asylum had been granted in the UK. A recent inspection report [37] (p. 8) on the provision and quality of accommodation highlighted issues of unsuitability based on poor property standards related to 'damp, dirt and vermin'.

On arrival at a host country, women are additionally traumatised when having to report the reasons for fleeing their country of origin by recounting their experience of violence and rape, more often than not, through an interpreter with no immediate psychological/emotional support or health interventions. Furthermore, some home office interviewers have been reported by women as not giving a full report or any acknowledgement of rape or violence having occurred, with many women also feeling that the quality of some interpretation services was inadequate [2].

The Refugee Council's Vulnerable Women's project report [38] on 153 asylum seekers in the UK indicated that 76% of women had been raped in their country of origin or in the UK, 22% had been sexually abused and 9% threatened with some form of sexual violence or abuse whilst being detained in their home country. Many women, not only those seeking asylum and refuge, have feelings of shame related to sexual abuse and violence. Although more contemporary data exists about the number of possible incidents, many cases, because of the associated shame and fear of reprisal, may go unreported. These women also suffer the possibility of being excommunicated from their families and communities for fear of bringing shame on them as a result of the rape and consequent pregnancy. These feelings of isolation lead to depression and suicide ideation in many women.

9.8   Female Genital Mutilation

Asylum seekers from countries from the continent of Africa such as Egypt, Sudan, Eritrea and Somalia and the Middle East and parts of South East Asia have a higher probability of presenting with female genital mutilation (FGM). This is a cultural practice steeped in traditions and, as such, has no benefit either physical or psychological for the woman. Women who have undergone FGM often feel anger and shame [39]. The WHO acknowledged [40] FGM as a violation of an individual's human rights and called for an end to this practice; however, it still takes place, and in a few cases, asylum is sought on the grounds of having undergone FGM. In the UK, health- and social care professionals have a statutory duty [41] to report to the police any cases of FGM in girls under the age of 18. This is also stipulated by the professional regulatory and statutory bodies in relevant practice guidelines and is mandatory under the Serious Crime Act 2015. FGM poses problems for the management of pregnancy and subsequent labour and birth as it has been associated with risks such as obstructed labour, Caesarean section and postpartum haemorrhage.

9.9   Modern Slavery and Human Trafficking

The Global Slavery Index (GSI) [42] describes modern slavery as an umbrella term that encompasses forced labour, human trafficking (across and within borders) and slavery that includes forced marriage. Based on available data collected in 2016, the GSI estimates just over 40 million of people globally are modern slaves, approximately 70% of whom are women and girls. Countries with repressive governments have weak legislation and policies to deal with the issues of modern slavery, which impacts the definition of slavery and its subsequent measurement. Modern slavery is a human rights abuse. Within the UK, the Modern Slavery Act of 2015 [43] is clear in its definitions of slavery and servitude.

Human trafficking involves the forced recruitment and travel of a victim either across country borders or within a country for exploitation. The United Nations Office on Drugs and Crime (UNODC) report of 2016 [44] estimated that women (51%) and children (28%) are the predominant victims of human trafficking. The National Crime Agency [45] offers categories of exploitation related to human trafficking that include organ harvesting, domestic servitude, forced labour and sexual exploitation. 99% of the victims trafficked for sexual exploitation are women and girls [44].

Some people may make claims for asylum when already living in the UK. These rare cases may be women who have been the victims of human trafficking for the specific purpose of exploitation linked to modern slavery as mentioned above. The process of seeking asylum in such cases is fraught with more difficulties, as the documents they need to provide (bank statements, council tax notice, tenancy agreements) may not exist in their name or be inaccessible to them, as they are held by their captor, thereby delaying their claim to asylum.

The National Crime Agency [45] leads the Modern Slavery Human Trafficking Unit (MSHTU), too. This is a multi-agency organisation that works alongside many UK government departments, including the Border Force and Immigration Enforcement teams, the police force as well as charities to protect and safeguard people in such situations. Any suspected case of modern slavery or human trafficking initially needs to be reported to the local police force. The MSHTU provides a single point of contact to support anyone working with, and for, people who may have been trafficked.

Victims of modern slavery and human trafficking suffer with the consequences of violence, sexually transmitted infections and a host of physical and psychological trauma because of their abuse. If there are such concerns related to any pregnant woman or anyone else you may encounter, then reporting of such suspicions is imperative and may help to alleviate suffering and exploitation and save lives.

9.10   Psychological Health and Wellbeing

Many women continue to suffer the psychological consequences of their trauma, long after they have been offered refuge and resettled in the host country. The trauma may result from a myriad of persecution experiences ranging from grief from the death of family and friends, violence, torture, rape and the migration journey through to the processes associated with resettling in the host country. There is a slow and gradual emergence of research on the mental health of asylum seekers and refugees. When compared to the host population, they have higher levels of mental health disorders such as anxiety attacks, depression and post-traumatic stress disorder (PTSD) and present with higher levels of suicide risk.

Poor mental health and psychological stress may present in many ways, and these are dependent on the cultural beliefs about mental health held by the individual woman. Some express depressive symptoms as feelings of sadness. Diagnoses of a mental health condition may also be viewed as a stigma [46], so some women may somatise their psychological symptoms describing them as headaches, or bodily aches and pains. Anxiety disorder symptoms may include extreme worrying, described as 'over-thinking', restlessness and excessive fear of strangers. Irritability, insomnia and fatigue are also commonly experienced. Symptoms of depression may also include insomnia, as well as persistently low and/or labile moods, lethargy and a general loss of motivation and interest in daily activities. Changes in weight, commonly weight loss, is also associated with depressive symptoms. Suicide ideation is commonly experienced and demonstrates a severe form of depression carrying a very high risk of suicide, as some plans may have been made about how to end their life. The symptoms of PTSD may include intrusive thoughts and vivid memories of past traumas. A heightened state of awareness and suspicion may be evident too in the form of sensitivity to noises or withdrawal from strangers or environments [47].

The precursors of these impacts on mental health are experienced whilst still in the home country either as a direct result from factors such as natural disasters, wars, persecution or having witnessed acts of violence and death. Understandably, poorer mental health status has been recorded in asylum seekers who have experienced such traumas prior to seeking asylum [48].

The uncertainty of their situation in seeking asylum is another contributory factor for poor mental health. The journey to escape may not have been without danger, with the added risks of experiencing violence or subjugation en route. The initial feelings of hope on arrival in a host country may quickly diminish due to the complexity of the asylum application process, coupled with the insecurity of either being granted asylum or deported. Language barriers, location and quality of accommodation, navigating new systems to access health- and social care, as well as adapting to living amongst new communities, and possibly experiencing different hostilities all add to the individual's mental stress burden.

Psychological and mental stress is still experienced once asylum has been granted and refugee status achieved. Stress arises from a sociological perspective in the form of acculturation [49]. Acculturation relates to the processes of trying to integrate with host communities, which pose challenges related to finding jobs, managing finances, living in unfamiliar areas, getting to grips with transport and utility services and the experience of discrimination. Acculturation has implications on the refugee's sense of personal identity and levels of self-esteem impacting their ability to understand how they fit in to the community, society and country that has offered them refuge.

Support systems, such as family, friends and the same cultural/religious communities, which can have a positive effect on mental wellbeing, either are completely lacking or become inconsistent and transient when women are housed in different areas. The fragility of these informal support systems, coupled with limited access to engage with formal mental health services, has a negative effect on a woman's ability to manage and understand the symptoms she may be experiencing, consequently impacting her resilience [50] and further exacerbating the stresses she may be experiencing. A woman's ability to make sense and adapt to different situations (resilience) will have a direct impact on any children she currently has or may have [51]. There is a greater risk of deepening depressive symptoms during pregnancy, something which any health professional should always be mindful of.

9.11 Conclusion

This chapter offered an outline of some of the issues faced by women seeking refuge in the UK, hopefully increasing awareness that becoming a refugee is no easy task and definitely not one that is sought through choice, more through a matter of survival, a basic human instinct. Some of the trauma that women have suffered remains with them for life, and it is only through a compassionate and sensitive approach to their care that we may begin to address some of the myriad of issues they face as they hope to build a new life for themselves and their family.

References

1. Universal Declaration on Human Rights. https://www.un.org/en/universal-declaration-human-rights/
2. Clayton G, Crowther T, Kerr J, Sharrock S, editors. Through her eyes: Enabling women's best evidence in UK asylum appeals. London: NatCen Social Research; 2017, Editor: Matt Barnard
3. Refugee Council. https://www.refugeecouncil.org.uk/information/refugee-asylum-facts/the-truth-about-asylum/
4. International Organisation for Migration; 2019. https://www.iom.int/key-migration-terms
5. UNHCR; 2016. https://www.unhcr.org/en-us/news/latest/2016/3/56e95c676/refugees-migrants-frequently-asked-questions-faqs.html
6. World Bank. Moving for prosperity. Global migration and labor markets. Policy research. Report. Washington: International Bank for Reconstruction and Development/The World Bank; 2018. https://doi.org/10.1596/978-1-4648-1281-1
7. UKGov.com. The process of seeking asylum. https://www.gov.uk/claim-asylum
8. Baillot H, Connelly E. Women seeking asylum: safe from violence in the UK?; 2018. http://www.asaproject.org/uploads/Safe_from_violence_in_the_UK._ASAP-RC_report_.pdf
9. Refugee Council. http://www.asylumineurope.org/reports/country/united-kingdom/reception-conditions/housing/types-accommodation
10. Feldman R. When maternity doesn't matter. Dispersing pregnant women seeking asylum; 2013). https://www.refugeecouncil.org.uk/information/resources/when-maternity-doesnt-matter-dispersing-pregnant-women-seeking-asylum/
11. National Asylum Support Service How to claim. https://www.gov.uk/asylum-support/how-to-claim
12. UNHCR Asylum in the UK. https://www.unhcr.org/asylum-in-the-uk.html
13. Maternity Action. https://maternityaction.org.uk/advice/asylum-seekers-financial-support-and-housing/
14. Bulman M. Thousands of asylum seekers and migrants wrongly denied NHS health care; 2017. https://www.independent.co.uk/news/uk/home-news/asylum-seekers-migrants-wrongly-denied-nhs-healthcare-cancer-doctors-phil-murwill-a7672686.html
15. Redman EA, Reay HJ, Jones L, Roberts RJ. Self-reported health problems of asylum seekers and their understanding of the national health service: a pilot study. Public Health. 2011;125:142–4. https://doi.org/10.1016/j.puhe.2010.10.002.

16. Oliver C. Country case study on the impacts of restrictions and entitlements on the integration of family migrants: qualitative findings. Oxford: Centre on Migration, Policy and Society (COMPAS) University of Oxford; 2013. https://www.compas.ox.ac.uk/2013/pr-2013-impacim_uk_qualitative/
17. UKDH NHS entitlements: migrant health guide. Advice and guidance for healthcare practitioners on the health needs of migrant patients. https://www.gov.uk/guidance/nhs-entitlements-migrant-health-guide#introduction
18. Home Office: Immigration rules https://www.gov.uk/guidance/immigration-rules/updates
19. Cheng I-H, Drillich A, Schattner P. Refugee experiences of general practice in countries of resettlement: a literature review. Br J Gen Pract. 2015;65(632):e171–6. https://doi.org/10.3399/bjgp15X683977.
20. National Institute for Health and Clinical Excellence Guidelines; 2010.
21. NICE Pregnancy and complex social factors: service provision overview. 2010. https://pathways.nice.org.uk/pathways/pregnancy-and-complex-social-factors-service-provision#content=view-node%3Anodes-coordinated-care-plan-and-information-sharing
22. Mother and babies: reducing risk through audits and confidential enquiries across the UK (MBRRACE-UK) November 2018. Lessons learned to inform maternity care from the UK and Ireland Confidential Enquiries into Maternal Deaths and Morbidity; 2014–16 Maternal, Newborn and Infant Clinical Outcome Review Programme.
23. Asif S, Baugh A, Wyn Jones N. The obstetric care of asylum seekers and refugees women in the UK. Obstet Gynaecol. 2015;17:223–31. https://doi.org/10.1111/tog.12224.
24. Heslehurst N, Brown H, Pemu A, Coleman H, Rankin J. Perinatal health outcomes and care among asylum seekers and refugees: a systematic review of systematic reviews. BMC Med. 2018;16:89. https://doi.org/10.1186/s12916-018-1064-0.
25. Aldridge RW, Nellums LB, Bartlett S, Barr AL, Patel P, Burns R, Hargreaves S, Miranda JJ, Tollman S, Friedland JS, Abubakar I. Global patterns of mortality in international migrants: a systematic review and meta-analysis. Lancet. 2018;392:2553–66. https://doi.org/10.1016/S0140-6736(18)32781-8.
26. Withers M, Kharazmi N, Lim E. Traditional beliefs and practices in pregnancy, childbirth and postpartum: a review of the evidence from Asian countries. Midwifery. 2018;56:158–70. https://doi.org/10.1016/j.midw.2017.10.019.
27. Lang-Baldé R, Amerson R. Culture and birth outcomes in Sub-Saharan Africa; a review of literature. J Transcult Nurs. 2018;29(5):465–72.
28. Hemmings S, Jakobowitz S, Abas M, Bick D, Howard LM, Stanley N, Zimmerman C, Oram S. Responding to the health needs of survivors of human trafficking: a systematic review. BMC Health Serv Res. 2016;16:320. https://doi.org/10.1186/s12913-016-1538-8.
29. Owens C, Dandy J, Hancock P. Perceptions of pregnancy experiences when using a community-based antenatal service: a qualitative study of refugee and migrant women in Perth, Western Australia. Women Birth. 2016;29:128–37. https://doi.org/10.1016/j.wombi.2015.09.003.
30. Scott J, Mullen C, Rouhani S, Kuwert P, Greiner A, Albutt K, Burkhardt G, Onyango M, VanRooyen M, Bartels S. A qualitative analysis of psychosocial outcomes among women with sexual violence-related pregnancies in eastern Democratic Republic of Congo. Int J Mental Health Syst. 2017;11:64. https://doi.org/10.1186/s13033-017-0171-1.
31. Novik D. Sit back and listen—the relevance of patients' stories to trauma-informed care. N Engl J Med. 2018;379(22):2093–4.
32. Reeves E. A synthesis of the literature on trauma-informed care. Issues Ment Health Nurs. 2015;36(9):698–709. https://doi.org/10.3109/01612840.2015.1025319.
33. Skjelsbæk I. Victim and survivor: narrated social identities of women who experienced rape during the war in Bosnia-Herzegovina. Feminism Psychol. 2006;16(4):373–403. https://doi.org/10.1177/0959353506068746.
34. Kinyanda E, Musisi S, Biryabarema C, Ezati I, Oboke H, Ojiambo-Ochieng R, Were-Oguttu J, Levin J, Grosskurth H, Walugembe J. War related sexual violence and its medical and psychological consequences as seen in Kitgum, Northern Uganda: a cross-sectional study. Int Health Hum Rights. 2010;10:28. http://www.biomedcentral.com/1472-698X/10/28

35. Revgev S, Slonim-Nevo V. Trauma and mental health in Darfuri asylum seekers: the effect of trauma type and the mediating role of interpersonal sensitivity. J Affect Disord. 2019;246:201–8. https://doi.org/10.1016/j.jad.2018.12.024.

36. Allotey P, Reidpath D. The health of refugees: public health perspectives from crisis to settlement. 2nd ed. e-book; 2018.

37. Bolt D. An inspection of the Home Office's management of asylum accommodation provision. HMSO; 2018.

38. Refugee Council. Vulnerable women's project: https://www.refugeecouncil.org.uk/?s=Vulner able+women%27s+project

39. Recchia N, McGarry J. "Don't judge me": narratives of living with FGM. Int J Hum Rights Healthcare. 2017;10(1):4–13. https://doi.org/10.1108/IJHRH-10-2016-0016.

40. WHO Eliminating female genital mutilation. https://www.who.int/reproductivehealth/publica-tions/fgm/9789241596442/en/

41. Nursing and Midwifery Council; 2018 https://www.nmc.org.uk/standards/code/female-genital-mutilation-cases/

42. The Global Slavery Index. https://www.globalslaveryindex.org/

43. The Modern Slavery Act; 2015. http://www.legislation.gov.uk/ukpga/2015/30/contents/enacted

44. United Nations Office on Drugs and Crime. Global report on trafficking in persons; 2016. https://www.unodc.org/documents/data-and-analysis/glotip/2016_Global_Report_on_Traf-ficking_in_Persons.pdf

45. The National Crime Agency. https://nationalcrimeagency.gov.uk/

46. Alemi Q, James S, Montgomery S. Contextualizing Afghan refugee views of depression through narratives of trauma, resettlement stress, and coping. Transcult Psychiatry. 2016;53(5):630–53. https://doi.org/10.1177/1363461516660937.

47. Aoun A, Joundi J, El Gerges N. Post-traumatic stress disorder symptoms and associated risk factors: a cross-sectional study among Syrian refugees. Br J Med Pract. 2018;11(1):a1106.

48. Hameed S, Sadiq A, Din AU. The increased vulnerability of refugee population to mental health disorders. Kansas J Med. 2018;11(1):20–3.

49. Kartal D, Kiropoulos L. Effects of acculturative stress on PTSD, depressive, and anxiety symptoms among refugees resettled in Australia and Austria. Eur J Psychotraumatol. 2016;7:28,711. https://doi.org/10.3402/ejpt.v7.28711.

50. Pangallo A, Zibarras L, Lewis R, Flaxman P. Resilience through the lens of interactionism: a systematic review. Psychol Assess. 2015;27(1):1–20.

51. Donovan CL, Holmes MC, Farrell LJ, Hearn CS. Thinking about worry: investigation of the cognitive components of worry in children. J Affect Disord. 2017;208:230–7. https://doi.org/10.1016/j.jad.2016.09.061.

Perinatal Peer Mentoring, Sexual and Reproductive Health and Rights, and HIV

10

Angelina Namiba ⓘ, Longret Kwardem ⓘ,
Rebecca Mbewe ⓘ, Fungai Murau ⓘ, Susan Bewley ⓘ,
Shema Tariq ⓘ, and Alice Welbourn ⓘ

Abstract

This chapter describes the 4M Programme, a perinatal peer mentoring programme led by, with and for women living with HIV in the UK. It considers HIV and pregnancy both within a UK and global context, describing the epidemiology as well as policy and practice. We then outline the background development and principles of the 4M programme, before highlighting successes and challenges of the programme and discussing future development.

Keywords

HIV and women · Sexual and reproductive health and rights · Peer mentoring · Violence · Mental health · Women · Pregnancy · Mentor Mother

A. Namiba (✉) · L. Kwardem · R. Mbewe
Salamander Trust Associate, London, UK

4M Mentor Mothers Network (CIC), London, UK
e-mail: longret@4mmm.org; rebecca@4mmm.org

F. Murau
4M Mentor Mothers Network (CIC), London, UK
e-mail: fungaim@ids.ac.uk

S. Bewley
Department of Women's and Children's Health, Kings College London, London, UK
e-mail: susan.bewley@kcl.ac.uk

S. Tariq
UCL Centre for Clinical Research in Infection and Sexual Health, London, UK
e-mail: s.tariq@ucl.ac.uk

A. Welbourn
Salamander Trust Associate, London, UK
e-mail: alice@salamandertrust.net

© Springer Nature Switzerland AG 2021
L. Abbott (ed.), *Complex Social Issues and the Perinatal Woman*,
https://doi.org/10.1007/978-3-030-58085-8_10

10.1   Introduction

It is very important that women get this type of training and get together more [...] the large majority of women are still in the dark about these issues. (Mentor Mother)

We describe how women living with HIV in the UK have created and led a perinatal peer mentoring programme, called 4M (Fig. 10.1), which has now become an independent Community Interest Company (CIC)[1], called 4M Mentor Mothers Network CIC. The programme supports a network of women living with HIV, who have themselves gone through pregnancy whilst knowing they have HIV, to work voluntarily with health and social care providers. Each 'Mentor Mother' can form part of a multidisciplinary HIV antenatal care team, providing peer support to women living with HIV who want this.[2] Alternatively, they can work informally within their local communities, supported directly by the 4M programme team.

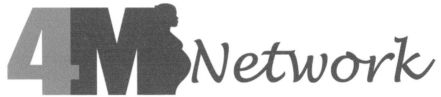

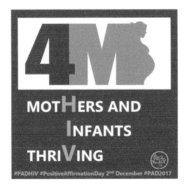

Fig. 10.1 The 4M logo and the 4M meme. The latter was developed by one of the programme's Mentor Mothers

---

[1] In the UK, a Community Interest Company (CIC) is a not-for-profit organisation.

[2] Several Mentor Mothers are linked to local HIV charities who can provide important ongoing support to Mentor Mothers in fulfilling their role. Other Mentor Mothers provide more informal peer support through their own networks.

We start by contextualising HIV and pregnancy, both within the UK and internationally, and describe the epidemiology and landscape of policy and practice. This is followed by a summary of the background development and principles of 4M. We highlight successes and challenges, discuss the programme's future development and end by highlighting the impact of the COVID-19 pandemic and lockdown on the lives of women living with HIV involved in the programme.

10.2   HIV and Pregnancy in the UK

There were approximately 29,700 women accessing HIV care in the UK in 2018 representing 31% of all adults living with HIV nationally [1]. Most women living with HIV in the UK are of Black African ethnicity and acquired HIV heterosexually.

Women living with HIV in the UK have long been recognised to face complex problems [2]. A report in 2018, from Sophia Forum and Terrence Higgins Trust, highlighted once more the relative neglect of women in the UK's HIV policy and service delivery, calling for renewed attention to key issues [3]. Almost half of the women surveyed reported living below the poverty line; over half had experienced violence as a consequence of their HIV status; and many described significant unmet needs around mental health, housing and immigration. Importantly, when considering the reproductive health and rights of women living with HIV, two-in-five respondents reported that HIV had influenced their decision about having children, and a third had avoided seeking healthcare through fears of discrimination [3].

An average of just under 1000 women with diagnosed HIV are currently reported as pregnant each year in the UK and Ireland; 66.4% were born in Africa, and around 15% were born in the UK or Ireland [4]. HIV can be acquired by infants in utero, during labour or through breastfeeding. This is known as *vertical transmission* of HIV. A combination of interventions including opt-out antenatal screening for HIV (with 97% uptake), use of HIV medication (ART) during pregnancy and for newborn babies and appropriate management of delivery and infant feeding has resulted in the extremely low vertical transmission rate of 0.27% in the UK [5].

The steep decline in vertical transmission of HIV both in the UK and globally is a key success story in HIV prevention. However, it is important to remember that pregnancy and early motherhood still remain a potentially challenging time for women living with HIV. Historically, the majority of pregnant women living with HIV in the UK learned about their HIV status when tested during that pregnancy. Life-changing medical diagnoses are particularly difficult to handle during pregnancy; it is difficult to grieve for the pre-diagnosis self at the same time as preparing for an important life event and worrying about the impact of disease and treatments. There may be an understandable time pressure and medical focus on the baby, to the detriment of positive, encouraging normalisation of mothering.

Nowadays, most women living with HIV in the UK know about their HIV status before conception. Nonetheless, complex HIV-associated psychosocial problems remain, potentially compromising maternal, infant and family wellbeing. For example, a 2018 national review of vertical transmissions identified issues including immigration, housing problems, intimate partner violence and other 'adverse social problems' as key contributing factors [6].Furthermore, a systematic review of HIV and perinatal mental health found a high prevalence of postnatal depression (30–53%) [7]. These psychosocial issues can be further exacerbated by interventions recommended to minimise the risk of vertical transmission. For example, current UK guidelines [8] recommend women to abstain from breastfeeding. However, for some women, this can lead to considerable emotional, social and financial cost, with reports of women living with HIV in the UK going without food to pay for formula milk [9, 10].

In the pre-ART era, up to 15–32% of babies who were breastfed for a year may have acquired HIV via this route. If women are taking lifelong ART, it looks as if transmission after birth is only 1–3% (over 6–12 months) [11], although this information has largely come from low-income countries. Advice in the UK has always previously been to avoid breastfeeding entirely. Current guidance still recommends formula feeding. However, it also states that if a woman wishes to breastfeed (and if she has an undetectable HIV viral load on ART), she should be supported to breastfeed exclusively (as opposed to mixed feeding) and be advised that a shorter duration of breastfeeding is associated with a lower risk of HIV transmission. In this situation, healthcare providers are recommended to monitor the mother and baby's viral load closely.

It is unknown how much lower the rate of transmission is among those women in high-income countries who adhere to treatment well, whose viral load is undetectable, who exclusively breastfeed for 6 months and who have regular testing. It may be a small number per thousand, or closer to zero. The long-term effects of ART on the baby via breast milk are also uncertain. In contrast to the UK, the World Health Organization (WHO) recommends that women living with HIV should breastfeed for at least 12 months and that this may continue for up to 24 months or longer (similar to the general population) whilst being fully supported for ART adherence [12, 13]. The WHO recommendation recognises the major role of breastfeeding in reducing infant and child mortality (especially in settings where formula feeding is not safe, feasible or affordable) and improving long-term health outcomes. These differences in guidance, all based in evidence, create difficult 'trade-offs' which should be discussed and individualised plans made. Many women in middle- and low-income countries can safely provide formula milk and may prefer to do so and many women in high-income countries cannot afford formula milk and/or may also prefer to breastfeed.

A 2020 4M advocacy brief on infant feeding sets out 4M members' own perspectives on the pros and cons of different methods of feeding their babies [14]. In particular, it includes the benefits of breast feeding and the drawbacks of formula feeding (most of which are missing from current BHIVA guidance) and includes women's own perspectives, so that other women living with HIV can feel empowered to make a more informed choice about infant feeding.

10.3   The Historical Global Context: From 'Elimination of Mother-to-Child-Transmission (eMTCT)' to Ensuring Sexual and Reproductive Rights (eSRHR)

In the earliest years, HIV was generally assumed only to affect men who had sex with men. Initially, few researchers or clinicians initially paid attention to its effects on women. This led women living with HIV to storm the stage of the International AIDS Conference in 1992, demanding that the conference should also recognise that HIV affects women [15]. Through this activism, the International Community of Women (ICW) living with HIV was born [16].

Policymakers can sometimes seem unconcerned by, or have limited awareness of the negative stereotypes created about women living with HIV, which obscure the realities of their complex lives. As knowledge of heterosexual and vertical transmission of HIV grew, women's pregnancies became a focus of attention for the biomedical community. Women, healthcare workers and society at large were concerned about women's potential to 'infect' (itself a loaded word) [17] their unborn babies with HIV. The prevalence of HIV 'in' pregnant women became the measure by which countries were listed in global HIV monitoring. In many countries, forced and coerced sterilisation of women living with HIV became widespread [18, 19], as did (and does) forcible HIV testing by healthcare workers even if official guidance indicates it is voluntary [20].

Historically, before ART became widely available, women were told not to breastfeed and to have caesarean sections. Over the years, these measures, combined with routine roll-out of maternal ART during pregnancy, have all contributed to global declines in vertical transmission rates. WHO now clearly recommends breastfeeding and normal vaginal delivery, with elective caesarean section only when needed, provided a woman is stable on ART. However, some women in middle- and low-income countries still report that they are pressured by health workers to have caesarean sections and not to formula-feed. Both these practices have considerable financial implications, quite apart from physical or emotional ones. Further, women who do not start or continue ART face the prospect of being described as having 'failed' to adhere, and labelled as 'lost to follow-up' or 'defaulters', with limited discussion about *why* they might not wish (or be able) to attend clinic after delivery, even if they attended whilst pregnant [21, 22]. In some centres, there is still open criticism and abuse of the women concerned, who often feel bullied out of care [13, 23].

This framing of pregnant women and new mothers as potential vectors of disease, rather than as women in their own right, is ethically challenging. It can feel dehumanising for women to be viewed merely 'as a means to an end' rather than 'an end in themselves'. Matters were further worsened in 2011 with the publication of the United Nation's 'Global Plan to Eliminate Mother to Children Transmission of HIV and Keep their Mothers Alive', soon known as the 'elimination plan' [24]. WHO 2016 guidelines on ART use was similarly unhelpful [25]. The rights of women living with HIV to voluntary, confidential and informed choice regarding sex, contraception, choices around pregnancy care and quality of life in general received only fleeting mention in both documents. Furthermore, the role of violence, both at home and in healthcare settings, as a treatment access barrier was entirely overlooked [16].

10.4   The Stereotype of 'Bad Mothers'

The image of pregnant women as troublemakers who need to be controlled, and who cannot be trusted to make 'good' informed choices for themselves, is long-standing. It is not confined to women living with HIV. The BBC journalist Kate Adie, herself adopted at birth, has described how badly women and their babies born outside socially accepted norms have been treated for centuries [26]. Her book encompasses many examples, including the original foundlings' hospital (for babies whose mothers either could not or were not allowed to keep them) [27]; the Ireland's Magdalena Sisters' convents for 'fallen' girls; and the treatment of women and children from traveller communities. Law professor Dorothy Roberts has described how racially minoritised women are often stigmatised and devalued as mothers due to racial stereotypes of being 'unfit'. These are enacted through racist welfare policies and the disproportionate criminalization of Black, Indigenous and other women of colour for relatively minor infractions, such as drug use in pregnancy [28]. Childbirth with HIV is perhaps the most recent example of an enduring, unacceptable, societal prejudice towards women and babies deemed to exist outside the straitjacket of prevailing social norms [29].

Such public attitudes are reinforced by medical training that has historically focused on biomedical approaches to women in their pregnancies, often removing all social context and women's feelings and agency [30]. This is exemplified in the historical illustration below (Fig. 10.2), used in a doctor-turned-anthropologist's

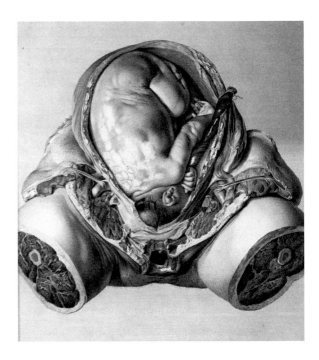

Fig. 10.2 A graphic example of how a woman's womb and baby have long been presented as disconnected from the rest of her body, both literally and metaphorically, in medical textbooks. Sinclair notes how there is great detail and that the image is detached from both the rest of the body and from any other context

analysis of 'the making' of doctors in a London teaching hospital [31]. Whilst Sinclair clarified that medical training has advanced considerably, biomedical prioritisation of infant wellbeing over the health and rights of individual women still holds true. In the management of HIV and pregnancy, the tendency to date has been an almost exclusive focus on prevention of vertical transmission.

10.5 HIV and Pregnancy: Towards a More Holistic, Women-Led Approach

Recent years have seen the UK's national professional HIV organisation, the British HIV Association (BHIVA), advocate a more holistic and woman-centred approach to HIV and pregnancy. The updated guidelines on management of HIV in pregnancy and postpartum do now explicitly recognise the psychosocial challenges women may experience during pregnancy, recommending a multidisciplinary approach, including peer support [7]. There has also been more recent discussion in general around the importance of healthcare providers being trained in 'trauma-informed' or 'trauma-aware' care [32].[3] However, women still face stigma in healthcare settings [33],[4] and mental health issues and intimate partner violence (IPV) remain common [34]. The first study of IPV amongst women living with HIV in the UK was published a little before [35] global research was taking place [36]. However, it was well after domestic violence was first measured in maternity and genito-urinary medicine clinics in the UK [37, 38]. The support of midwives and clinicians in recognising and addressing these challenges is critical in improving care for women living with HIV in the UK.

The WHO now provides clear guidance on the health and rights of women living with HIV across the lifespan in its 'Consolidated Guideline on the Sexual and Reproductive Health and Rights of women living with HIV' [11]. Containing new recommendations and good practice statements, it was based on a global survey led by women living with HIV on their values and preferences [39]. Using a house model (Fig. 10.3), this survey depicted women's multifaceted lives and recognised the importance of addressing all elements in order to provide effective support. These represent a shift from the idea of 'woman as vessel' and the sole focus on the HIV status of the infant in global research, policy and practice, towards the often-neglected quality of life of women and girls. The survey showed how much women living with HIV experience violence and mental health issues, either starting at or

---

[3] Canadian Activist and Indigenous elder Valerie Johnson points out that the term 'trauma-aware' may be more appropriate. This is because an individual may not feel able to share information about the traumas she/he may have experienced with a service provider. Yet the service provider should be trained nonetheless to be aware that traumas may have taken place and should take the possibility of these into account in the care given the individual concerned, especially with regard to her/his capacity to trust in and access services.

[4] The reported attribution of blame to women for their babies' deaths in Shrewsbury and Telford Hospital NHS Trust, reported in 2020, is another example of this (https://www.ockendenmaternityreview.org.uk/first-report/)

Fig. 10.3 The 'house' model shows the bedrock of respect, support and safety that is needed for women living with HIV to flourish and then be able to care for others [39]

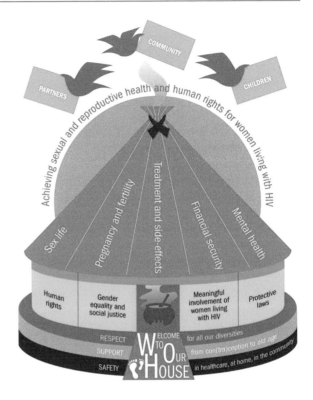

exacerbated by their diagnosis [31, 40]. Further research, again led by women living with HIV, has shown how much these factors can act as a treatment access barrier, if not addressed [41]. We also know that these issues increase in pregnancy and are linked to poor maternal and infant outcomes [42].

It takes a radical shift, often from female leaders, to see women as 'ends' in themselves (with their own intrinsic outcomes) rather than merely as 'means' (instrumental for others' outcomes), or even as both. Women living with HIV have their own dreams, aspirations, rights and *agency*. When cared for well, they are best placed to look after their own health and wellbeing, to take medication and to look after their families [43].

Since the HIV pandemic began, women living with HIV globally have done much to support themselves. Indeed, the whole HIV peer support self-help movement reportedly grew from the influence of the Boston Women's Health Collective and its groundbreaking 1971 self-help manual, *Our Bodies Ourselves* [44].

Peer support is recognised as a bedrock of self-help therapeutic responses in many varied contexts [45]. In the UK, a formal peer support model by women living with HIV began with the founding of the Positively Women charity in 1987 [46]. There is good evidence of the efficacy of perinatal peer support in improving psychosocial, health and behavioural outcomes in pregnancy [47]. Specifically in HIV, it has been shown to have positive psychosocial impacts, with improvements in clinical outcomes in randomised controlled trials [48, 49].

The first UK grassroots charity-led Mentor Mother programme led by, and for, women living with HIV was the London-based 'From Pregnancy to Baby and Beyond' hosted by Positively UK. Angelina Namiba, one of this chapter's co-authors, and a co-Director of 4M Mentor Mothers Network CIC, created the original programme. The programme linked Mentor Mothers to healthcare providers and HIV charities. The programme trained women living with HIV as Mentor Mothers, so that each could work as part of a multidisciplinary team of health- and social care providers to support women living with HIV throughout their pregnancies. Each Mentor Mother was also linked to a local HIV charity, to receive ongoing support. The programme ran successfully from 2010 to 2015, when funding ceased [50]. A formal evaluation demonstrated positive multidimensional impacts on women's emotional wellbeing whilst leading to personal growth among Mentor Mothers themselves [41].

10.6   The Conception of 4M

The 4M Programme, coordinated by Salamander Trust (a global HIV charity), stands for 'My health, My choice, My child, My life'. It is an innovative, peer-led training programme, responding to the psychosocial challenges experienced by women living with HIV during the perinatal period (from pre-conception planning through to childbirth and early motherhood). Its primary aim is to build a sustainable network of women living with HIV across the UK, who are trained as peer support workers (Mentor Mothers).

Approximately 65% of women living with HIV in the UK and Ireland who are pregnant live outside London [5]. These women may face particular challenges through a lower concentration of HIV and other relevant support organisations locally. Therefore, building upon previous successes, Salamander Trust aimed to expand the Mentor Mother programme across the UK from 2016. Women living with HIV were trained in accordance with the UK's National Standards for Peer Support in HIV [51]. The programme is still led and delivered by women living with HIV and, in July 2019, became registered as its own independent CIC, with the same women as its directors, all of whom are Black African migrants. From inception, 4M has had a steering group comprising women living with HIV, researchers and clinicians, providing managerial and strategic guidance.

4M conducted eight national training workshops in partnership with regional HIV charities in 2016. These were the Sussex Beacon, (Brighton); Body Positive (Bournemouth); Terrence Higgins Trust (Cardiff); Positive East (Essex); Hwupenyu Health and Wellbeing (Glasgow); Black Health Agency (Leeds); Faith in People with HIV (Leicester); and George House Trust (Manchester).

The two-day training included clinical and psychosocial aspects of pregnancy and HIV and creative writing sessions. Full details are available in our national training manual [52]. The creative writing elements were included to stimulate trainees' reflections on their own journey to motherhood. It was vital to offer a safe space in which Mentor Mothers could reflect upon their personal experiences whilst gaining skills and confidence to share these with their peers.

Our subsequent objective in 2017 was to scale up the programme. 4M conducted a national 'Training of Trainers' workshop with 14 Mentor Mothers. This aimed to build women's skills and capacity to facilitate 'The Pregnancy Journey' workshop for other women living with HIV and to be recognised as qualified trainers. Components included The Pregnancy Journey; Incorporating the UK Standards of Peer Support into mentoring roles; Creative Writing; Understanding Our Sexual Health and Reproductive Rights; and an Introduction to Monitoring and Evaluation.

Following this workshop, the Mentor Mothers created their own national network. In 2018, the successful 4MNet network was formed via WhatsApp, supplemented with emails when required [53]. A webinar series was also launched (see below).

In October 2019, the 4M Mentor Mothers Training of Trainers manual was launched online. This received widespread acclaim and (as of June 2021) has been downloaded 46 times for use or review by various organisations internationally (including the UN). Their stated locations for use include East, West and Southern Africa, South and South East Asia, China, North America, Sweden, Russia, the Caribbean and the UK [54].

In autumn 2020, the programme published an advocacy brief about the focus of its work, calling for a shift from 'eMTCT' to 'eSRHR', which stands for 'ensuring the sexual and reproductive health rights' of women living with HIV throughout pregnancy [55]. This brief was followed by two policy briefs. The first set out the pros and cons of breastfeeding versus formula feeding, and the second described the multiple challenges experienced by 4M members and the women they support during the 2 COVID-2019 lockdown in 2020 [14, 56].

This network of determined, resilient women living with HIV provides a UK-wide community forum of mutual support, information exchange and encouragement. It facilitates Mentor Mothers' ongoing work in supporting other women living with HIV across the UK throughout pregnancy whilst also generating evidence that can be used to inform policy.

10.7 How This Programme Differs from Other Peer-Led HIV Mentor Mother Programmes

4M is grounded by a woman-centred approach with rights-based and gender-equitable principles and is thus closely aligned with the WHO Consolidated Guideline [32].A fundamental element is that if and when women living with HIV decide to have a baby, the best way to support them and their baby is to uphold women's own rights, enabling them to feel happy, healthy and safe throughout conception, pregnancy, delivery and postpartum.

In other countries, HIV Mentor Mother programmes have been initiated by healthcare providers and/or related organisations led by clinicians. Whilst these may have been beneficial, they sometimes overlooked principles of sustainable community development practice, including:

(i) Recognition of the power of grassroots-led ownership of initiatives to effect changes in attitudes towards an issue
(ii) Recognition of voluntary activism of those most affected by an issue as a key coping strategy, thereby:
(iii) Constituting a form of therapeutic response in itself
(iv) The importance of not undermining voluntary, community-led initiatives through well-intended, top-down, 'professionalised' interventions

As externally driven interventions often lack local knowledge or insights, they can result in the collapse of local, small-scale, voluntary initiatives. Key to the success of all peer-support programmes is that they are created and led by those who share lived experience. The powerful reassurance that 'I am not alone', combined with detailed local knowledge and a willingness to develop context-appropriate solutions through team work, shape and drive their sustainability.

Since inception, 4M has embedded formal evaluation into the programme, employing a 'bottom-up' methodology of participatory action and empowerment peer research [57], where the 4M participants are active researchers in the programme, working alongside academic evaluation team members. This approach, which ensures meaningful involvement of those most affected by an issue, is gaining traction in the world of HIV. Recent operational research with UNAIDS and partners shows policymakers, researchers and programme practitioners how they can use such participatory approaches to strengthen and expand the evidence base around violence against women and HIV [58, 59].

The 4M programme lead evaluator (LK) is a peer researcher and steering group member, involved in the programme from the start. Two of the 14 women trained in the October 2017 Trainers workshop have now joined the evaluation team. This has enabled peer researchers to develop professionally. We have used both formal and more participatory mixed-methods approaches, combining quantitative questionnaires with qualitative interviews (and other methods) with Mentor Mothers and local HIV charities, to enable 4MNet members to identify their own indicators of programme success and to measure these, along with challenges [53, 54].

10.8   4M Results so far

In the first 2016 round, 46 women aged 22–67 in eight locations across mainland UK were trained; the majority of women were Black African, reflecting the epidemiology of HIV in women in the UK. All Mentor Mothers anonymously rated training components as 'good' or 'excellent' immediately after completion. Likewise, nearly 90% reported improvements in both knowledge about HIV and pregnancy and confidence in action planning.

On returning to participants 6 months later, all 21[5] who responded reported that 4M had resulted in durable improvements in knowledge of HIV and pregnancy, and

---

[5]At this time, several of the organisations that hosted the training workshops were facing huge funding constraints, and two had to close down. So this response rate was better than hoped for.

action planning, as well as increased self-confidence, reduced isolation and a greater sense of community. Almost three-quarters expressed interest in becoming trainers themselves.

In qualitative evaluation, conducted through telephone interviews, Mentor Mothers described developing empathy through personal sharing, increasing their sense of belonging and reducing isolation. They highlighted programme leads' sensitivity and reflection, which contributed to an inclusive and safe space (Box 10.1).

Box 10.1 4M Feedback from Mentor Mothers and Clinicians

'It feels good as a woman living with HIV to be able to give the right information.' (Mentor Mother)

'I have learnt a lot from the training, I am able to practise in my own life.' (Mentor Mother)

'Training has given me hope that there is more to life than worrying about am I going to die and what am I going to do?' (Mentor Mother)

'I have gone through all the stages the sickness the help, bullying the stigma, I have gone through all those and then and not being able to talk about it [...] It can help anyone else as it has helped me. Find my feet again, I have started working and I never thought I will be able to do that.' (Mentor Mother)

'I've also done some clips for the health students in a university, so they invited me to record a clip that they will be using whenever they are training [...] before the Mentor Mother training, I don't think I would've be able to do that but now, I've got into that level where I feel I'm okay to share.' (Mentor Mother)

'The 4M TOT [...] was an incredibly valuable experience, it was an opportunity to process the past, open very guarded doors, get angry, and be with my pain. Time is so precious, and time to belong, to experience empathy and support, to feel a sense of togetherness allowed me to become strong, in a more powerful way than resilience.' (Mentor Mother)

'The power of peer support at this point in an HIV journey is enormous. The 4M project, with a programme of work delivered from and for people living with HIV with real, lived experience adds a new dimension [...] the visibility of women living with HIV demonstrates to others the possibility of living openly and well with HIV, something that many people have never believed to be a reality [...] this is a programme that makes a difference. Because it is co-produced between women living with HIV and their clinicians it is particularly powerful and relevant. It makes a real difference.' Jane Anderson (Clinician and Steering Group Member)

'Having worked in HIV clinics with and without peer mentors readily available, I have seen the positive effects that they can make to women providing psychological support, reducing isolation, challenging stigma and empowering them to make educated decisions about their own health [...] the

outputs have been presented both nationally and internationally [...] 4M has also been asked to train other healthcare professionals such as midwives about HIV and has contributed to consultations regarding the new BHIVA Guidelines for Pregnant women.' Rageshri Dhairyawan (Clinician and Steering Group Chair)

Mentor Mothers particularly valued the creative writing component and its potential to draw out resilience and increase self-confidence in delivering peer support. The participants' creative writing was compiled into a booklet aptly named 'The Songs of Experience' [60]. This was shared publicly in March 2018 to celebrate International Women's Day (Box 10.2).

Box 10.2 Creative Writing by One Mentor Mother from the Training of Trainers Workshop
Susie Onion
I'm carrying the whole world over my shoulder as a colourful coat. The strength of my feet shows in the mountains and the hill ground I've walked, stumbled, upon.

Despite the clearly visible layers I wear and the tears, it's difficult to be seen by others. There are so many voices, dreams, visions, hopes, songs.

I have the strength to stand to be seen. I'm still standing, peeling off layers and layers, getting fresh as an onion.

At the time of evaluation, five Mentor Mothers had provided peer support to eleven women following training. Barriers to this included Mentor Mothers' social circumstances and health issues and lack of robust links with local clinics and support services.

The HIV charities who set up workshops in partnership with 4M rated the training as valuable, engaging and relevant. However, they identified key challenges in implementation and sustainability, such as limited training time, volunteer retention and lack of awareness of the Mentor Mother programme among services and clinics [61].

10.9   Parallel Processes

Although not covered here, the 4M training has appealed to others in low- and middle-income settings, because of its effectiveness and relatively low cost. Training workshops have been conducted with partners PIPE Trust (Kenya) and the Uganda Network of Young People living with HIV [62]. They are currently looking for further funding to expand these pilot programmes. As described above, the manual has also been downloaded by various organisations in a range of countries internationally.

10.10 The Future of 4M

In summary, despite significant biomedical developments in HIV treatment during pregnancy, women continue to encounter psychosocial challenges. As the HIV pandemic has evolved, so have approaches to pregnant women living with HIV. Grounded in the same woman-centred approach with gender-equitable and rights-based principles as the WHO 2017 guideline, the 4M programme is a highly valuable, sustainable and acceptable perinatal peer support programme led by and for women living with HIV, fostering resilience and self-efficacy among Mentor Mothers. It is also in line with the ethos of UK standards for peer support. In developing a national network of trained Mentor Mothers, 4M has built an invaluable national resource to complement the clinical care of women living with HIV during pregnancy and early motherhood. 4M continues to raise awareness within clinics of the existence of Mentor Mothers, through dissemination of our 2018 advocacy report [63], so that health- and social care professionals can refer clients who may require such support.

In order to sustain the programme, especially during the ongoing COVID-19 pandemic which places both practical and economic constraints on the delivery of services, we now seek funds to reshape the training component so it can be delivered online. Early data have shown that COVID-19 and lockdown measures have had a detrimental effect on maternal mental health [64]; this is likely to be even more pronounced in the context of women living with HIV who often have other co-existing psychosocial challenges. Therefore, programmes, such as 4M, which prioritise support to pregnant women and new mothers are in need more than ever.

Additionally, we have conducted a webinar training series that is archived online for others to access. 4MNet members decided the topics collectively. As of December 2020, there were 14 archived webinars. Topics include updates on national and international guidance such as WHO's Consolidated Guideline on SRHR of women living with HIV, the importance of trauma-informed care, infant feeding, COVID and pregnancy and other topics; quality of life for women living with HIV; how best to talk to children and significant others about HIV status; immigration issues; welfare and benefits; confidence around attending meetings and being an effective patient representative; report and abstract writing and submission and related conference tips and strategies; links between SRHR, violence against women and girls, mental health and HIV; HIV, pregnancy and COVID-19; HIV health inequalities with a focus on perinatal care; digital literacy; and social media for change.[6]

With sustainability as a core principle, we are conscious that young women who acquired HIV vertically are now transitioning from paediatric to adult care. The 4M model will be a useful resource to young women and to healthcare professionals managing this group. Mentor Mothers have been appointed to serve as steering committee members on the Collaborative HIV Paediatric Study (CHIPS).[7] This will

---

[6] To access the full webinar series, see https://vimeo.com/user128708330.

[7] The CHIPS study is investigating the long-term health of young people who were born with HIV or acquired it in early childhood (http://www.chipscohort.ac.uk/).

ensure that the principles of the 4M model are carried through the continuum of care as girls living with HIV enter adulthood.

Although 4M was designed specifically for women living with HIV, it is adaptable to other areas of support for women in pregnancy, some of which are also addressed in this book. These include mental health conditions, domestic violence, incarceration, sex work, drug use, sexual orientation, gender identity, disability and immigration issues. 4M is making links with organisations outside the HIV sector, providing peer support to women during pregnancy. Building these partnerships will allow for shared learning, as well as creating opportunities for further work more broadly on perinatal peer support by, with and for socially marginalised women.

In conclusion, 4M highlights the potential for peer-support programmes to foster personal and professional growth of the women involved, as they (re)discover and hone their own strengths and resilience. The main threat to the success of programmes like ours is the ongoing funding challenge experienced by all third sector organisations in the current political economic, social, technological, legal and environmental context and exacerbated by the impact of COVID-19 [65, 66]. We hope that books like this will shine a light on how much is possible, with relatively little financial input, if only women are supported to enable their dreams to be realised (Box 10.3): throughout their pregnancies and beyond.

Box 10.3 Some Top Tips for Best Practice When Caring for Women Living with HIV

Top Tips

Here are some suggestions for best practice when caring for women living with HIV:

Assume the pregnant woman cares about her own and her baby's health.

If the woman has anxieties about confidentiality, it may take a whilst to build trust.

Be aware of the powerful feelings of shame that keep many issues hidden and the fear anyone in a position of authority might invoke.

Anger is often a mask for unmet fears, hurts and needs and a response to past or current traumatic events; peer supporters may help to unpack and resolve these.

Offer *all* pregnant women (not just those with HIV or complex social issues) basic written information about how to get help with domestic violence, alcohol and drugs, previous trauma, legal support with immigration, food banks, etc.

Be careful to use non-judgemental language.

Find positive, empowering, inclusive, solution-focused language such as 'you are not alone', 'it's so great that you are looking after yourself and your baby by being here', or 'how do you feel we can best support you?'

Avoid being nosy about how the HIV was acquired. Is this question really necessary for the woman's own health and/or that of her baby? If so, explain how.

Consider what conversations are relevant to present care and you can do something about (e.g. offering non-judgemental support or resources that help).

Be aware of local and national HIV support services (such as perinatal peer mentoring), and consider referral when appropriate.

Acknowledgements This chapter has been prepared with the support of the 4M Steering Group, whose members are Rageshri Dhairyawan, Shema Tariq, Jane Anderson, Susan Bewley, Pat Tookey, Gill Gordon, Vicky Johnson and Alison Wright; the 4M Programme, Longret Kwardem, Rebecca Mbewe and Angelina Namiba; and the Salamander Trust, Alice Welbourn. The 4M programme has been funded by MACAIDS Fund and ViiV Healthcare. Former 4M Programme member Nell Osborne designed and led the Creative Writing workshops.

Declaration of Conflicting Interests The authors declared no potential conflicts of interest with respect to the research, authorship and/or publication of this article.

Funding The authors received no financial support for the research, authorship and/or publication of this article.

References

1. Public Health England. HIV in the United Kingdom: Towards Zero HIV transmissions by 20302019 report. London: Public Fitness England; 2019, https://assets.publishing.service. gov.uk/government/uploads/system/uploads/attachment_data/file/858559/HIV_in_the_ UK_2019_towards_zero_HIV_transmissions_by_2030.pdf
2. Doyal L, Anderson J. HIV-positive African women surviving in London: report of a qualitative study. Gender Dev. 2006;14(1):95–104.
3. Sophia Forum and Terrence Higgins Trust. Women and HIV: invisible no longer. In: A national study of women's experiences of HIV; 2018. http://sophiaforum.net/wp-content/ uploads/2018/04/Invisible-No-Longer-full-report-of-a-national-study-of-women-and-HIV.pdf.
4. National Study of HIV in Pregnancy and Childhood. Obstetric and paediatric surveillance data. Population, policy and practice programme. UCL Great Ormond Street, Institute of Child Health; June 2020 update. https://www.ucl.ac.uk/nshpc/resources/biannual-data-update-slides
5. Peters H, Francis K, Sconza R, Horn A, Peckham C, Tookey P, Thorne C. UK mother to child HIV transmission rates continue to decline: 2012-2014. Clin Infect Dis. 2016; https://academic.oup.com/cid/article/64/4/527/2623961
6. Peters H, Thorne C, Tookey PA, Byrne L. National audit of perinatal HIV infections in the UK, 2006-2013: what lessons can be learnt? HIV Med. 2018;19(4):280–9. https://onlinelibrary. wiley.com/doi/epdf/10.1111/hiv.12577
7. Kapetanovic S, Dass-Brailsford P, Nora D, Talisman N. Mental health of HIV-seropositive women during pregnancy and postpartum period: a comprehensive literature review. AIDS Behav. 2014;18:1152–73.
8. Gilleece Y, Tariq S, Bamford A, Bhagani S, Byrne L, Clarke E, et al. British HIV Association guidelines for the management of HIV in pregnancy and postpartum (2020 3rd interim update); 2020. Available at https://www.bhiva.org/file/5f1aab1ab9aba/BHIVA-Pregnancy-guidelines-2020-3rd-interim-update.pdf

9. Tariq S, Elford J, Tookey P, Anderson J, de Ruiter A, O'Connell R, Pillen A. "It pains me because as a woman you have to breastfeed your baby": decision-making about infant feeding among African women living with HIV in the UK. Sex Transm Infect. 2016; https://doi.org/10.1136/sextrans-2015-052224.

10. National AIDS Trust. Policy briefing: access to formula milk for mothers living with HIV in the UK; 2017. https://www.nat.org.uk/publication/policy-briefing-access-formula-milk-mothers-living-hiv-uk

11. Bispo S, Chikhungu L, Rollins N, Siegfried N, Newell M. Postnatal HIV transmission in breastfed infants of HIV-infected women on ART: a systematic review and meta-analysis. J Int AIDS Soc. 2017;20(1):21,251. https://www.ncbi.nlm.nih.gov/pmc/articles/PMC5467610/

12. See https://www.who.int/elena/titles/hiv_infant_feeding/en/. Accessed 15 December 2020.

13. WHO. Consolidated guideline on sexual and reproductive health and rights of women living with HIV. Geneva: World Health Organization; 2017. http://apps.who.int/iris/bitstream/handle/10665/254885/9789241549998-eng.pdf;jsessionid=EF82749F7C5991A077DFFCB18519A5C3?Sequence=1

14. 4M Mentor Mothers Network CIC & Salamander Trust. Position paper on infant feeding for women living with HIV; 2020. Available at https://4mmm.org/wp-content/uploads/2020/12/4M_Breastfeeding_PaperAugust2020.pdf

15. Women's Networking Zone. Amsterdam revisited—26 years on—back to the birthplace of the International Community of Women living with HIV: The Women's Networking Zone: standing on the shoulders of giants. Women's Networking Zone; 2018. http://salamandertrust.net/wp-content/uploads/2018/07/WNZ_2018_Standing_on_the_shoulders_of_giants.pdf

16. http://www.icwglobal.org/our-organization/history

17. Dilmitis S, Edwards O, Hull B, Margolese S, Mason N, Namiba A, et al. Language, identity and HIV: why do we keep talking about the responsible and responsive use of language? Language matters. J Int AIDS Soc. 2012;15(Suppl 2):17,990.

18. Paxton S. Positive and pregnant: how dare you—a study on access to reproductive and maternal health care for women living with HIV in Asia [Internet]. Asia Pacific Network of People living with HIV; 2012. http://www.unaids.org.cn/pics/20130222153427.pdf

19. Southern Africa Litigation Centre. African Commission on Human and Peoples' Rights Condemns Involuntary Sterilisation of Women Living with HIV In Africa. Southern Africa Litigation Centre [Internet]. Southernafricalitigationcentre.org; 2013 [cited 7 May 2015]. http://www.southernafricalitigationcentre.org/2013/11/12/african-commission-on-human-and-peoples-rights-condemns-involuntary-sterilisation-of-women-living-with-hiv-in-africa/#

20. Olowokere AE, Adelakun OA, Komolafe AO. Knowledge, perception, access and utilisation of HIV counselling and testing among pregnant women in rural communities of Osogbo town, Nigeria. Aust J Rural Health. 2018;26:33–41. https://doi.org/10.1111/ajr.12368. https://onlinelibrary.wiley.com/doi/full/10.1111/ajr.12368

21. Orza L, Bass E, Bell E, Crone E, Damji N, Dilmitis S, et al. In women's eyes: key barriers to women's access to HIV treatment and a rights-based approach to their sustained well-being. Health Hum Rights J [Internet]. 2017;19(2):155–68. [cited 2 July 2018]. https://cdn2.sph.harvard.edu/wp-content/uploads/sites/125/2017/12/Orza.pdf

22. Bewley S, Welbourn A. Should we not pay attention to what women tell us when they vote with their feet? AIDS. 2014;28(13):1995.

23. UN. Agenda for Zero discrimination in health-care settings. UN 2017. http://www.unaids.org/sites/default/files/media_asset/2017ZeroDiscriminationHealthCare.pdf

24. UN. Global plan towards the elimination of new HIV infections among children by 2015 and keeping their mothers alive 2011-2015 [Internet]; 2011. http://www.unaids.org/sites/default/files/media_asset/20110609_JC2137_Global-Plan-Elimination-HIV-Children_en_1.pdf

25. WHO. Consolidated guidelines on the use of anti-retroviral drugs for treating and preventing HIV infection. 2nd ed. [Internet]; 2016. http://apps.who.int/iris/bitstream/10665/208825/1/9789241549684_eng.pdf?Ua=1

26. Adie K. Nobody's child. London: Hodder; 2006.

27. https://www.coram.org.uk/about-us/our-heritage-foundling-hospital

28. Roberts D. Killing the black body: race, reproduction and the meaning of liberty. Vintage; 2000.
29. Welbourn A. Desires denied: sexual pleasure in the context of HIV. In: Jolly S, Cornwall A, Hawkins K, editors. Women, sexuality and the political power of pleasure [Internet]. London: Zed Press; 2013. [cited 23 September 2018]. https://www.zedbooks.net/shop/book/women-sexuality-and-the-political-power-of-pleasure/.
30. Cohen Shabot S, Korem K. Domesticating bodies: the role of shame in obstetric violence. Hypatia. 2018;33(3):384–401.
31. Sinclair S. Making doctors: an institutional apprenticeship. Oxford: Berg; 1997. https://www.bloomsbury.com/uk/making-doctors-9781859739501/
32. Hall D, Fraser K. Becoming trauma-informed, 4M Webinar no. 8, 2019, Salamander Trust. Available at https://vimeo.com/showcase/6971206/video/361065776
33. Ferraro C, Benton L, Lut I, Hudson A, Kirwan P, Jefferies J, Delpech V, Okala S, Sseruma W, Mbewe R, Morton J, Valiotis G, Kunda C, Jamal Z, Reeves I, Nelson M, Ross M, Wolton A, Cardwell H, Sharp L. Experiences of stigma among people living with HIV accessing care through the National Health Service. HIV Med. 2016;17(1). Poster 50. https://www.bhiva.org/file/mdhwnvegnimke/abstractbook2016.pdf
34. Orza L, Welbourn A, Shentall L, Sachikonye M, Bewley S, Strachan S. "Listen to us, learn from us, work alongside us": UK findings from a global participatory survey; 2016. http://salamandertrust.net/wp-content/uploads/2017/02/BHIVA_Poster_2016_ukwomen_Salamander_Sophia.pdf
35. Dhairyawan R, Tariq S, Scourse R, Coyne K. Intimate partner violence in women living with HIV attending an inner city clinic in the UK: prevalence and associated factors. HIV Med. 2012;14(5):303–10. https://onlinelibrary.wiley.com/doi/full/10.1111/hiv.12009
36. Orza L, Bewley S, Chung C, Crone E, Nagadya H, Vazquez M, et al. "Violence. Enough already": findings from a global participatory survey among women living with HIV. J Int AIDS Soc [Internet]. 2015;18(Suppl 5). https://www.ncbi.nlm.nih.gov/pmc/articles/PMC4672459/
37. Bacchus L, Mezey G, Bewley S, Haworth A. Prevalence of domestic violence when midwives routinely enquire in pregnancy. BJOG. 2004;111(5):441–5. https://doi.org/10.1111/j.1471-05 28.2004.00108.x.
38. Loke W, Bacchus L, Torres C, Fox E. Domestic violence in a genitourinary medicine setting—an anonymous prevalence study in women. Int J STD AIDS. 2008;19(11):747–51. http://journals.sagepub.com/doi/10.1258/ijsa.2008.008117
39. Orza L, Welbourn A, Bewley S, Crone E, Vazquez M. Building a safe house on firm ground: key findings from a global values and preferences survey regarding the sexual and reproductive health and human rights of women living with HIV [Internet]. Salamander Trust; 2015. http://salamandertrust.net/resources/BuildingASafeHouseOnFirmGroundFINALreport190115.pdf
40. Orza L, Bewley S, Logie C, Crone E, Moroz S, Strachan S. et al., How does living with HIV impact on women's mental health? Voices from a global survey. J Int AIDS Soc [Internet]. 2015;18(Suppl 5). https://www.ncbi.nlm.nih.gov/pmc/articles/PMC4672402/
41. Orza L, Bass E, Bell E, Crone E, Damji N, Dilmitis S, et al. In women's eyes: key barriers to women's access to HIV treatment and a rights-based approach to their sustained well-being. Health Hum Rights J. 2017;19(2):155–68. [cited 2 July 2018]. https://cdn2.sph.harvard.edu/wp-content/uploads/sites/125/2017/12/Orza.pdf
42. Making Waves Network. Obstetric violence, respectful maternity care, and women and adolescent girls living with HIV—Upholding our SRHR as essential during COVID-19 and beyond; December 2020. https://makingwaves.network/2020/12/08/obstetric-violence-respectful-maternity-care-and-women-and-adolescent-girls-living-with-hiv-upholding-our-srhr-as-essential-during-covid-19-and-beyond/
43. Beres L, Narasimhan M, Robinson J, Welbourn A, Kennedy C. Non-specialist psychosocial support interventions for women living with HIV: a systematic review. AIDS Care. 2017;29(9):1079–87.
44. Boston Women's Health Collective, editor. Our bodies ourselves: a book by and for women. 2nd ed. New York: Boston Women's Health Collective; 1976.

45. Side by Side Research Consortium. Developing peer support in the community: a toolkit; 2017. https://www.mind.org.uk/media/17944275/peer-support-toolkit-final.pdf
46. http://positivelyuk.org/about/
47. National Voices, Nesta. Peer support: what is it and does it work?: National Voices, London; 2015.
48. McLeish J, Redshaw M. 'We have beaten HIV a bit': a qualitative study of experiences of peer support during pregnancy with an HIV Mentor Mother project in England. BMJ Open. 2016;6(6):e011499.
49. Richter L, Rotheram-Borus MJ, Van Heerden A, Stein A, Tomlinson M, Harwood JM, et al. Pregnant women living with HIV (WLH) supported at clinics by peer WLH: a cluster randomized controlled trial. AIDS Behav. 2014;18(4):706–15.
50. http://positivelyuk.org/pregnancy/
51. National Standards for Peer Support in HIV. 2017. http://hivpeersupport.com/
52. Namiba A. Mentor mother trainers' guide, volumes 1 and 2; 2019. Salamander Trust and 4M Mentor Mothers Network CIC.
53. Kiersten Hay K, Kwardem L, Welbourn A, Namiba A, Tariq S, Coventry L, Dhairyawan R, Durrant A. "Support for the supporters": a qualitative study of the use of WhatsApp by and for mentor mothers with HIV in the UK. AIDS Care. 2020;32(suppl 2):127–35. https://doi.org/1 0.1080/09540121.2020.1739220.
54. Salamander Trust, 4M Manual Endorsements. 2019.
55. From elimination of MTCT to ensuring SRHR. Advocacy brief; 2020. Salamander Trust and 4M Mentor Mothers Network CIC.
56. Confinement: women, HIV and pregnancy during the 2020 COVID-19 lockdown in the UK. 2020, 4M Mentor Mothers Network CIC and Salamander Trust.
57. IIED. Participatory learning and action. Website. https://www.iied.org/participatory-learning-action-pla
58. Action linking initiatives on violence against women and HIV everywhere, ALIV(H)E framework. Salamander Trust, Athena, UNAIDS, AIDS Legal Network, Project Empower, HEARD, University of KwaZulu-Natal; 2017. http://salamandertrust.net/wp-content/uploads/2017/11/ALIVHE_FrameworkFINALNov2017.pdf
59. Hale F, Bell E, Banda A, Kwagala B, van der Merwe L, Petretti S, et al. Keeping our core values ALIV[H]E. Holistic, community-led, participatory and rights-based approaches to addressing the links between violence against women and girls, and HIV. J Virus Eradication [Internet]. 2018;(3). [cited 23 September 2018]. http://viruseradication.com/journal-details/Keeping_our_core_values_ALIV[H]E._Holistic,_community-led,_participatory_and_rights-based_approaches_to_addressing_the_links_between_violence_against_women_and_girls,_and_HIV/
60. Salamander Trust. Songs of Experience; 2018. https://issuu.com/salamandertrust.net/docs/4mnet_tot_manchester_creativewritin
61. Kwardem L, Anderson J, Welbourn A, Namiba A, Tariq S, Tookey P. 4M, my health, my choice, my child, my life: developing a national network of mentor mothers to support women living with HIV through pregnancy—a 6 month evaluation PE18/12 European AIDS Clinical Society EACS; 2017. http://resourcelibrary.eacs.cyim.com/mediatheque/media.aspx?mediaI d=34397&channel=28172
62. 4M+: Peri-natal Peer Mentoring Programme for women living with HIV. Advocacy Brief about the 4M+ Programme. Salamander Trust; 2018.
63. Salamander Trust. 4M advocacy brief—May 2018. Salamander Trust; 2018. https://issuu.com/salamandertrust.net/docs/salamandertrust4madvocacybrieffinal
64. Hessami K, Romanelli C, Chiurazzi M & Cozzolino M COVID-19 pandemic and maternal mental health: a systematic review and meta-analysis, J Matern Fetal Neonatal Med, 2020;1–8, https://doi.org/10.1080/14767058.2020.1843155
65. HIV Psychosocial Network. Ten years after: an 'austerity audit' of services and living conditions for people living with HIV in the UK, a decade after the financial crisis. The HIV Psychoso-

cial Network; 2018. https://hivpsychosocialnetworkuk.files.wordpress.com/2018/11/10-years-after-final.pdf.

66. Salamander Trust, et al. Fund what works: fund community-led women's rights organisations for an effective, ethical and sustainable response to HIV. The WHAVE Podcast Paper #1; 2020. https://salamandertrust.net/wp-content/uploads/2019/02/20200331_The_WHAVE_paper1_Funding_Final.pdf

Maternity Service Provision for Deaf Women and Women with Hearing Impairment

11

Paulina E. Sporek de Lacerda

Abstract

Effective and individualised antenatal care and parent education, safe expert care in labour, and competent care postnatally are the fundaments of contemporary midwifery practice. This chapter is designed to enable midwives, midwifery lecturers, student midwives, and other maternity healthcare practitioners to gain understanding of issues concerning deafness in order to improve the maternity care offered to deaf and hearing impaired women.

Keywords

Deaf women · Hearing impairment · Pregnancy · Sexual and reproductive health and rights · Equality · British sign languages · Lip reading · Deaf nest project

11.1 Introduction

Hearing impairment remains the most sensory deficit in the human population, with the problem currently affecting over 250 million people in the world [1]. It is worth noting that some of the consequences of hearing impairment include the incapability to interpret and make a proper speech and reduced ability to converse. Deaf people are therefore limited to use either sign language or lip reading to engage with other people. Deaf individuals face considerable obstacles; they are frequently educated below their capacity, employed below their capability, and viewed negatively by the hearing world because they are deaf. The fact that being deaf is viewed negatively in our society creates complicated interactions between deaf people and the hearing professionals with whom they come in contact.

P. E. Sporek de Lacerda (✉)
UCLPartners, London, Greater London, UK

© Springer Nature Switzerland AG 2021
L. Abbott (ed.), *Complex Social Issues and the Perinatal Woman*,
https://doi.org/10.1007/978-3-030-58085-8_11

Hearing loss has significant personal and social costs. The barriers deaf families encounter include discriminatory health and social support services and limited access to information. Those barriers not only erect restrictions to participation in the normal life of the community but also place limits on women's psycho-emotional wellbeing. This being a significant drawback to the research since the "Saving Lives, Improving Mothers' Care" report [2] has again identified the links between social exclusion and vulnerability and adverse pregnancy outcomes. Additionally, there is little literature available on providing maternity care to deaf parents. The lack of relevant literature suggest that deafness and pregnancy are two concepts rarely considered together. Despite the most recently available statistic which shows a dramatic increase in hearing loss, little has been said or done in relation to pregnancy and childbirth. That necessitates a serious discussion in regard to how maternal services can be streamlined to ensure the highest level of satisfaction for the deaf women and women with hearing impairment.

11.2 What Is Deafness?

Deafness is referred to as the partial or total inability to perceive sounds. Symptoms of deafness can be classified into those that are mild, moderate, severe, or profound. Profoundly deaf individuals cannot hear anything, and hence, they communicate by use of sign language or understanding through lip reading. It is therefore essential to understand that there is a variation between hearing loss and deafness; hearing loss is the reduction in the ability to hear sounds in a usual way, while deafness occurs when someone cannot understand speech through hearing even when there is an amplification of sound.

11.2.1 How Does Hearing Occur?

Hearing depends on a series of complex steps that change sound waves in the air into electrical signals. Sound waves enter the outer ear and travel through the ear canal, which leads to the eardrum which vibrates from the incoming sound waves and sends these vibrations to three tiny bones in the middle ear. These bones in the middle ear amplify the sound vibrations and send them to the cochlea in the inner ear. Once the vibrations cause the fluid inside the cochlea to ripple, a traveling wave forms along the basilar membrane. Hair cells change the vibrations into electrical signals that are sent to the brain through the hearing nerve which turns it into a sound that we recognise and understand. Therefore, the ear itself does not hear; it just receives sound waves which are transmitted as impulses to the brain. The brain interprets these as sound.

11.2.2 What Are Causes of Hearing Loss and Deafness?

There are two main types of hearing loss, depending on where the problem lies (Fig. 11.1):

- *Sensorineural hearing loss* is caused by damage to the hair cells inside the inner ear or damage to the hearing nerve. This kind of hearing loss is permanent.
- *Conductive hearing loss* is caused by a blockage of the air passageway through the ear. This hearing loss can be temporary or permanent.

It is also possible to have both types—this is known as **mixed hearing loss**.

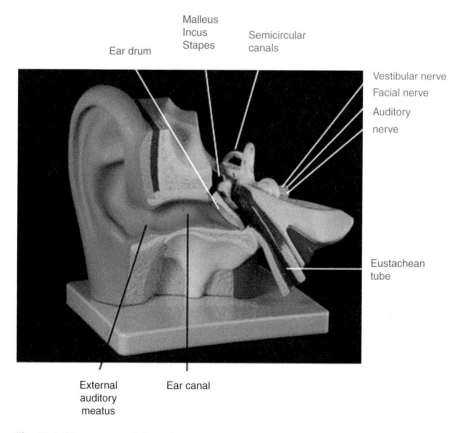

Fig. 11.1 Human ear model sample anatomy of the external, middle, and inner ear for didactic illustration to patients at the Brazilian Ear Institute

In addition to these, It is worth knowing other possible causes, and these are:

Noise-induced hearing loss	This is caused by prolonged exposure to excessive levels of noise, for example, in noisy workplaces or while listening to loud music. It can also be caused by extremely loud bursts of sound. Some people experience tinnitus as the first sign that their hearing has been damaged by noise
Genetic hearing loss	This type of deafness is present at birth. In the UK, about 1 in 1600 children is born moderately to profoundly deaf because they inherit a mutated gene
Acquired deafness	This type of deafness occurs after birth and may be caused by: • *Outer ear conditions*: earwax build-up, otitis externa, exostosis • *Middle ear conditions*: otitis media, glue ear, chronic suppurative otitis media, otosclerosis, damaged ossicles, perforated eardrum • *Inner ear and balance problems*: ear infections, benign paroxysmal positional vertigo, Meniere's disease • *Disease*: measles, mumps, meningitis
Otosclerosis	Otosclerosis is a condition that mainly affects the tiny ossicles (bones) in the middle ear. Twice as many women as men are diagnosed with otosclerosis. Some women report that the condition gets worse during pregnancy, and it is thought that this may be due to the high concentration of the hormone oestrogen during pregnancy
Acoustic neuroma	This is a rare, slow-growing tumour that develops on the eighth cranial nerve—the nerve of hearing and balance

Reflective activity

Find out more about causes of deafness by accessing the Action on Hearing Loss website here: *www.actiononhearingloss.org.uk*

11.3   Medical Model Versus Deaf Culture

In matters regarding the deaf culture, there is always a debate about the medical versus the cultural view of deafness. Many people in the society view deafness as a pathological condition and hence regard it as an undesirable condition that is supposed to be stopped or avoided. There are three primary models used in the classification of deafness the medical, social, and cultural models. The models of deafness seek to provide an understanding of the condition. The application of a given model affects how the person who is suffering from the condition views the world.

11.3.1 Medical Model

The medical model is viewed to be a defect that should have been avoided or treated when it occurred. In most cases, it is usually a result of another health problem. Individuals under this model may use hearing aids or undergo surgeries that may assist in the restoration of their hearing. Based on the model, the person with the condition is viewed as disabled, a view that is avoided in the modern world. Emphasis is placed on the possible ways of rehabilitating the condition with the available medical interventions with little attention being given to the uniqueness of the person and the possibilities of improving the quality of life without necessarily applying medical rehabilitation techniques.

11.3.2 Social Model

In the social model, there is an emphasis on the social aspect of the condition. Based on this model, the person is described as being hard of hearing or deafened. The model appreciates that the person who has this condition needs intervention in order to improve the overall quality of life. This model stresses the essential aspect of education and rely training at a young age to enable deaf individuals to communicate with both non-hearing and hearing people. The education aims to enable those with hearing impairments to live in a society and achieve their full potential.

11.3.3 Cultural Model

Regarding the cultural point of view, deafness is embraced as an identity. Those who embrace deafness as an identity do not focus much on the disability aspect but instead the uniqueness in other traits that such an individual may process. For populations of the deaf people, unlike expectant parents with disabilities, expectant deaf parents, like those in any other language minority, commonly hope to have children just like themselves, with whom they can share their language, culture, and unique experiences. Members, who decide to commit to the deaf culture, use the sign language for communication. Under this model, individuals do not, in most cases, go to seek medical attention regarding the condition.

In self-identification in the deaf community, regarding the deaf person with an upper case letter "D" is taken to mean those who view their deafness as a cultural choice. On the other hand, those with the lower case "d" regard their deafness as a disability. Those referred to with the capital D identify as part of the deaf community, while those with a small "d" are deaf but generally not regarded to be part of the deaf community. Identifying the identity of the patient and the way he/she regards the condition is crucial in ensuring that the interventions offered do not conflict with the personal views.

Reflective activity

Think about your cultural identity. What does it mean to you? How do you see deafness? Write one word to describe it.

11.4 British Sign Language

British Sign Language is a form of language that is dependent on the use of body language, gestures, facial expressions, and hand movements to aid in communication (Fig. 11.2). Fingers are used to illustrate or show English alphabets and teaching various nouns like names of people, places, and objects [3]. In the BSL, a complete statement or scene can be communicated in one sign. Unlike oral communication where views are delivered each after another, sentences in oral communication are therefore longer than in a sign language. The language is mainly used by people with hearing impairment [4]. It is estimated that 24,000 people on the UK use British Sign Language (BSL). Sign language can vary from one country to

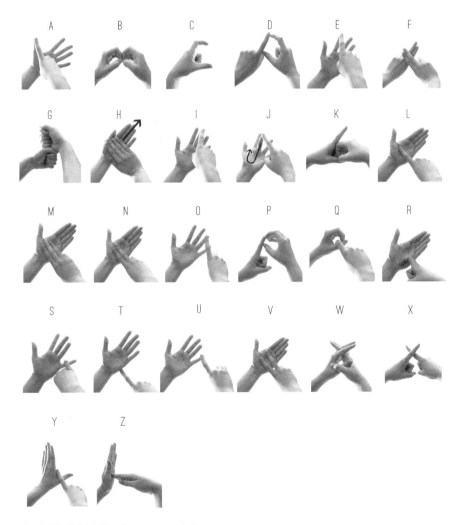

Fig. 11.2 British Sign Language alphabet

another. For example, there is a vast difference between the American and the British Sign Language.

For quite a long time, deaf people in the UK had been oppressed until a big campaign in 2003 where BSL was recognised by the UK government as an official minority language. This has led to increased funding for the needs of the communication of people who are Deaf and an increased awareness of the language which now has a similar status to that of other minority national languages such as Gaelic and Welsh.

Broadcasting channels in the UK use sign language to incorporate the deaf or as a way of providing information to them through programs specially made for them. The NHS choices website features 10 videos in sign language, of a possible 900 videos.

The application of BSL in the care of women who are deaf during delivery is dependent on the ability of both the patient and the midwife to communicate using this language. When the clinician is unable to use the language, an interpreter can be used to mediate the interaction. It is important for the midwife to address the patient just like in the usual care setting requirements. The interpreter has to be taken through the care needs of the patient since he/she is bound by confidentiality.

Practical activity

Using the British Sign Language alphabet, spell your full name.

11.5   Lip Reading

Lip reading is a technique used in communication whereby there is an interpretation of the movement of the lips, the face, and the tongue. In this technique, those communicating rely mostly on the image of the person who is talking to interpret what is being communicated. Lip interpretation depends on the lip reader's knowledge of a particular language, hence is more efficient when the reader is doing it in their first language. Lip reading is a crucial tool when communicating with a person when sounds may not be perceived mainly due to hearing loss.

Lip reading is, in most cases, meant for the deaf, but on the other hand, any average person is capable of reading lips and interpreting the information being given or communicated. For example, for infants who are learning on speech, they begin by studying their closest people lip positions and movement during communications.

In order to ensure adequate person-centred care for women with hearing impairment during the delivery process, it is crucial for the midwives to understand the possible ways of communication with the clients. Lip reading offers a good avenue through which the midwife can offer instructions during the process of delivery and ensure that the patient benefits from the best care possible based on the needs.

An important point to note during the application of the tool of communication is its effectiveness in the clinical setting. Since lip reading depends on the ability of the receiver to decode the information as the caregiver speaks, it is crucial to ensure that there is enough lighting. The source of light should also be preferably in front of the speaker since light from the back is only likely to cast a shadow and impair the interpretation of the message. The clinician should always ensure that the patient is attentive during the communication episode by taping her hand between the elbow and the wrist before the commencement of communication. It is worth noting that during delivery, the eyes of the mother are not always open. Alerting the patient before commencing with the communication episode helps ensure that there is no communication failure throughout the session. According to research, women with disabilities are at a higher risk of developing complications related to delivery. Unobstructed communication with the hospital staff, however, can help improve prognosis.

Things to remember when communicating with lip speakers

While using lip reading, various barriers may cause its inefficiency: an individual's commutation style may hinder lip reading. For example, if a person covers a part of the lips, it may be challenging to read their mouths and interpret what they could be saying.

Having a unique dialect or an accent may result in inefficiency in lip reading because with the uniqueness, they are likely to pronounce words differently from usual way.

Some people speak while their hands are on their mouth or while moving back and forth, and this may hinder lip readers from understanding, hence making the skills unreliable.

The length of a sentence can also lead to difficulties in lip reading due to the complexity of words.

Exaggerated speech patterns and failure to incorporate facial expressions may lead to difficulties in understanding lip reading, which requires a collaboration of all of them.

Background noise and the use of unfamiliar vocabulary while giving a speech may also act as a barrier for lip reading.

Practical activity

Practice lip reading from the distance when you are in a busy clinical setting.
• *What helps you to understand what is being said?*
• *What are the barriers?*
• *What could you do to improve the process?*

11.6   Statistics

Hearing loss is a major and growing public health issue, currently affecting more than 11 million people in the UK. Additionally, it is estimated that by 2035, there will be around 15.6 million people with hearing loss across the UK—that is one in five of the population.

Hearing loss has significant personal and social costs. There is a strong correlation between hearing loss and physical, emotional, mental, and social wellbeing. What evidence is available indicate poorer physical health among deaf people. The results from Action on Hearing Loss [5] research found that three in five (57%) respondents said that staff at GP surgeries, health centres, or hospitals had not asked about their individual communication needs. In addition, nearly two-thirds (64%) said they felt unclear about the information they have been given at their GP appointments [6]. The Ear Foundation estimates that, because of communication difficulties, people with hearing loss cost the NHS £76m in extra GP visits every year. Without access to a well-qualified communication professional, people who are deaf, in particular, are at risk of poor care and poor health. SignHealth estimates that the missed diagnosis and poor treatment of people who are deaf costs the NHS £30m every year.

The Equality Act 2010 and Disability Discrimination Act 1995 provide a clear legal foundation for providing access to healthcare for people with hearing loss. However, findings from research suggest that people with hearing loss still face challenges when accessing healthcare.

11.7 Barriers

The barriers that deaf women encounter during the prenatal care process include the lack of enough knowledge by the midwife on how to cater for their diverse needs as well as the inability for both parties to use the right communication tools. Additionally, there are huge barriers to access health services and lack of integration between them. Communication is the most serious barrier for deaf women and women with hearing loss. A British Sign Language interpreter is not always available to attend every antenatal, intrapartum, and postnatal appointment, yet communication plays a central role in underpinning informed consent and informed choice. In order to make informed choices, a woman needs accurate and accessible information. Iqbal (2004) [7] recognised that deaf parents are unable to access information, and this is mainly due to staff's inability to communicate in sign language or because of a lack of deaf awareness. Elaborating this theme, Price [8] utilises the idea that any communication barriers may compromise the quality of care. Other have followed a similar path when thinking about the importance of obtaining informed consent and ensure deaf women's rights and expectations are met under the Patient's Charter and Disability Discrimination Act (1995) [9].

11.8 The Results of the Study: No Sign of Support

Based on the study by Amanda O'Hearn (2006) [10] evaluating the experiences and satisfaction of deaf women with prenatal care, the results indicated that deaf women were less satisfied with the communication of the physician when compared to hearing women. The overall satisfaction with care was also lower for deaf women when compared to hearing women. The markers of satisfaction with the services provided for the deaf women included the provision of interpreter services during the times of consultation. On the other hand, hearing women had a higher number of visits for prenatal care with more information being offered to them during the prenatal visits by the attending physicians [10]. The research was qualitative in nature with the method of data collection being the provision of questionnaires to 23 deaf women and 32 hearing women. The questionnaires used were obtained from the modification of Omar and Schiffman's prenatal satisfaction measure.

Case Study

Rose is a 29-year-old first-time mum-to-be and profoundly deaf. She has been deaf since she was 3 years old and relies on lip reading.

Since finding out I am expecting a baby, I have come across so many more barriers. Deaf parents-to-be do not really have easy access to antenatal information. I cannot even book antenatal classes myself. I sometimes hate going to hospital appointments by myself as I have to constantly try and listen out for my name being called and concentrate on what the doctor is telling me. I sometimes think my eyes deceive me when I am trying to lip read and think is that me they are calling out or is it another Laura?! Sometimes I get up at the wrong time, and it is someone else they are calling out. I have once missed an appointment due to not hearing my name being called out.

After having my baby, I was on the ward, and my buzzer did not work, and I was told that the midwives were aware of my hearing loss as I was worried I would not be able to hear my baby cry at night. But they did not let me know when she was crying; I just simply did not sleep for 24hours! I do feel frustrated that deaf parents are not given accessible information. I would like to think that I have a support network around me available like hearing people have.

Reflective activity

Think about Laura's experience.

11.9   The Role of the Midwife in Maternity Service Provision

Midwives serve as autonomous practitioners; they behave like advocates for the women and aim to provide safe, quality, and evidence-based care for childbearing women and the newborn. There was never a time in the history of midwifery when the role of the midwife was more diverse than now. Deaf pregnant women are often neglected when accessing midwifery services [11]. The inequality is often a result of poor communication and women not receiving sufficient information regarding their pregnancy and childbirth. To extend control for such women over how they enjoy antenatal care, midwives have to understand the health disparities that may impact the access of healthcare services for these women. This is achieved by saving time to comprehend their concerns and adjusting their services and practices towards incorporating the unique needs of these women and their families. Midwives, therefore, have a task of learning how to use signs and other effective communication skills while providing care for deaf women. The caregivers should work towards fighting against barriers that affect women negatively during pregnancy and childbirth.

11.10   Choice and Control

Based on the Changing Childbirth report, the presence of emotional support and effective communication of expectant women improves the outcome of the pregnancy. When caring for the woman with deafness, the midwife is expected to offer the same assistance as to women with hearing ability [12]. For this to be possible, the midwife has to understand the best communication approach and create a friendly environment where the patient feels safe to air any concerns regarding the care given [13]. Interestingly, deaf women are now benefiting largely from the prospects of current information technology (IT) when accessing healthcare services. They proudly use mini-cams and text phones plus web facilities to increase their freedom of earning primary care [14].

Deaf cultural competency training for medical staff and midwives has in modern times improved skills in caring for deaf pregnant mothers, thus lowering the level of healthcare inequalities [15]. However, there is still a gap that midwives and nurses concerned with these women need to fill; they have to understand different backgrounds of deaf women with emphasis on the communication strategies they feel more comfortable with Middleton et al. [16]. There are different efforts made by individual countries in implementing feasible care units for women with disabilities more so in low- and middle-income countries. Universal primary care systems are therefore in need of experienced midwives, nurses, and doctors who will take the cases of deaf women seriously [17, 18].

11.11   Antenatal Period

11.11.1   Pregnancy Issues

In most care settings, the maternity care of deaf pregnant women is substandard mainly due to the lack of understanding on how to care for them and their diverse needs especially in regard to communication [19]. In order to ensure the maintenance of high-quality services for these women, the caregivers have to exchange information on what works best in such situations. It is also crucial to understand the specific needs of the deaf woman during the care process and shape the interventions to best suit the communication and care deficits of the patient [19].

Just like in the care of women with hearing ability, pregnant women with hearing impairment need care in regard to nutritional guidance, psychological care, and guidance on the substances that should be avoided during pregnancy. The midwife has to ensure that the client is adhering to the essential self-care approaches with the deficits noted being communicated to the patient in a manner that will enhance understanding [8]. The compliance to evidence-based care approaches is ensured by recognising the effective communication approaches such as the use of BSL and lip reading and offering specific instructions. It is crucial to managing the woman with hearing impairment just like the ones with hearing ability with the only adjustment being in the delivery of the necessary information regarding care. The patient's psychological health should also be evaluated and the necessary support offered in case of depression.

11.11.2 Parent Education

The first step in the care of the deaf pregnant woman in terms of education is to ensure a comprehensive assessment of the knowledge she has about the pregnancy and effective self-care approaches [13]. As the midwife, it is crucial to interact actively with the patient through writing or even an interpreter in order to have a comprehensive understanding of the level of understanding regarding the care process. When the midwife understands the level of knowledge of the deaf expectant woman, it becomes easier to commence with the education process starting from the known to the unknown. It is also crucial to ensure that the patient benefits from the maximum input of the clinician by ensuring that the most effective mode of communication is used. Whenever possible, the patient should be given supportive documents and pamphlets to enhance what has been taught during clinic visits. The pamphlets are also helpful since they can be adjusted to accommodate illustrative pictures which have shown to aid in the understanding of the content that has been taught [20].

The maintenance of the continuity in the education process for the pregnant woman with deafness can be ensured through the use of technological tools. An important tool in this care approach is the use of mobile phones [21]. The midwife can ensure that the client adheres to the right care approaches through supportive messages and online links to supportive documents on self-care. Even though the patient might be unable to use the technological tools verbally, it is possible to access documents regarding care and the latest evidence-based care approaches during the pregnancy. The application of technological tools in the education process can also be used to ensure that the patient does not miss out on any schedule antenatal care visits.

11.12 Intrapartum Period

11.12.1 Possible Issues

Based on a retrospective study exploring the pregnancy outcomes among deaf women in Washington State, 1987–2012 [22], it was noted that the chances of development of adverse pregnancy outcomes were similar between deaf pregnant women and women with hearing ability. The study also showed an increase in the number of days of hospitalisation of the women with deafness after delivery when compared to the control group. In caesarean birth, women with deafness had an increased chance of going through the procedure compared to non-deaf women. According to the study, deaf women have increased chances of a higher cost of care due to increased hospitalisation and increased chances of going through caesarean section [22]. The increased chances of longer hospitalisation and probability of going through operative delivery can be due to the existence of deficits in regard to the interpretation of the care needs of the deaf women by the caregivers [19].

The access to the right management processes is impaired by the lack of understanding of the specific patient needs. During delivery, the communication approaches that have been effective in antenatal care need to be adjusted. While the care of the pregnant woman with hearing ability involves verbally expressing the instructions during the process of birth, the care of the woman with hearing impairment requires skill and patience. In this instance, the patient may not be able to maintain eye contact with the clinician. As a result, approaches such as lip reading and the use of sign language become ineffective. In order to ensure adherence to the instructions during normal delivery, the midwife and the patient have to decide on the specific signs that will be used to direct the patient on the expected behaviour [13]. The clinician has to ensure that the patient understands the instructions during the time of delivery to ensure that avoidable complications are not encountered. The lack of coordination between the patient and the clinician causes a failure in the adherence to the best possible evidence-based management approaches [23].

11.12.2 Interpreter

The midwife should consider speaking directly to the woman rather not to the interpreter. She hence should sit or start at a position facing the woman, which will help maintain eye contact. For those that are in the lip reading category, simple English should be used, and the nurse should avoid having the mask on because it hinders lip reading. The midwife's patience is required because if the woman is tired or anxious, the service provider has to repeat the statements to ensure that the woman understands.

11.12.3 An Environment

A well-lit room should be used so that the woman can understand what the interpreter does or says. The midwife should speak normally, including facial expressions and gestures and ensure that all she says are things that she wants to be interpreted to the deaf woman. The reason for that is because the interpreter will interpret everything she says. When it is the interpreters turn, the speaker or rather the midwife should allow the interpreter to finish first; in most cases, the interpreter is usually some words behind the speaker.

11.12.4 Power of Touch

During labour, women in most cases have their eyes closed, this hence making it challenging to communicate with the deaf through sign language. In the effort to solve that, the midwife can reassure the woman by using touch, for example, tapping her arm for reassurance. In at least one maternity room, text phones should be installed to aid in communication when the woman gets anxious and unable to communicate.

11.13 Postnatal Period

11.13.1 Caring for the Baby

Mattresses that vibrate should be available in the postnatal ward. Such kind of service will help deaf women to know when the baby cries. In the case where the deaf women share a labour room with the rest, it is crucial to inform the others of her disability to ensure that they also give her the necessary attention whenever she needs it. It is vital to ensure that those women using hearing aids do not lie on the side, which covers the device hence preventing them from hearing.

11.13.2 Infant Feeding

The normal response of the child to distress including hunger is to cry [24]. For a midwife, it is important to ensure that the deaf woman can tell when the child is in distress and be able to differentiate when the distress is due to hunger or other environmental insults. The application of technological advancements has also made it easier for such mothers especially due to the ability to convert the crying of the infant to other forms of energy such as vibrations [25]. Depending on the level of hearing the loss in the patient, the midwife should ensure that there is adherence to the right breastfeeding schedule including exclusive breastfeeding for the first 6 months of life. In cases when the patient has no access to such tools, the clinician should help establish a favourable schedule of breastfeeding in order to maximise the possible gain of the child. Just like in the other points of care, the primary caregiver should offer recommendations that are in agreement with the preferences of the client.

11.14 Midwives Learning Needs

Midwives have for long earned recognition for their work of providing healthcare for deaf pregnant women. However, unlike in the past, modern midwives are finding the need to undergo special training to increase their knowledge more so when it comes to dealing with deaf mothers. As indicated by the RCM, it is the duty of midwives to create their practice by responding to the needs of these women and those of their families. Through learning and training, midwives are able to overcome prejudices, make informed decisions, and provide timely and carefully mediated healthcare in addition to communicating effectively. In Leicester, for instance, midwives are earning training on how to give sign language instructions to pregnant women as one way of effecting communication [26]. Academic institutions such as De Montfort University are offering course on the issues faced by the deaf—especially the new and future mothers.

11.15   What Is the Deaf Nest Project?

The Deaf Nest believes that understanding, respecting, and embedding diversity in maternity care have the potential to make a real difference to deaf women's experience of pregnancy and childbirth. The Deaf Nest Project is a vision of maternity services where every deaf parent has full access to services, an excellent childbirth and pregnancy experience, and the information to make informed choices. The Deaf Nest Project aims to improve deaf users' personal experience, equality of access, and choice and control over maternity care. Pregnancy and motherhood are major life events for all women, not least for deaf women. Nevertheless, they need to be accepted and supported in their choice to become parents and to be cared for and treated like every other woman. Until recently, little has been known about the deaf world in relation to pregnancy, and there appears to have been limited promotion of values and views except deaf people themselves. Additionally, deaf women and hearing-impaired mothers are a very small minority among the many thousands of hearing mothers that midwives see every day. Despite that, demand is no less urgent because it is not widespread—after all, each mother is an individual, and midwives must adopt their care accordingly.

Reflective activity

Check the Deaf Nest Project website, and find out more about pregnancy and deafness. Record at least one thing that you learned that you could bring into practice (*www.deafnest.com*).

11.16   Conclusion

In caring for pregnant women with deafness, the midwife has to adjust accordingly to enable the client to fully benefit from evidence-based care. Identifying the specific needs of the deaf woman and the best way to communicate forms the first step in the care process. The use of sign language, lip reading, written instructions, and an interpreter comes in handy in ensuring that the woman adheres to the ideal care practices. The midwife should also ensure continuity in the care process from the antenatal care to the care after delivery. It is also important for the midwife to ensure that all the decisions arrived at during the care process are guided by the choices of the client. As the primary caregiver, it is crucial to ensure that everyone in the care continuum contributes to the management of the patient.

Acknowledgements   I primary thank all the deaf parents who took part in the project; without you, there would be no project—thank you for sharing your experiences; it was an honour and privilege to hear your emotional stories. Thank you to SignHealth for all your support, encouragement, and commitment to me and the project. Special thanks to Dr. Jacque Gerrard who provided me with valuable feedback on the project and for insight, support, and inspiration.

References

1. Gordon KA, Papsin BC. Special edition on unilateral deafness and hearing loss: an introduction and overview. 2019:1–2.

2. Knight M, Bunch K, Tuffnell D, Jayakody H, Shakespeare J, Kotnis R, Kenyon S, Kurinczuk JJ, editors. On behalf of MBRRACE-UK. Saving lives, improving mothers' care—Lessons Learned to Inform Maternity Care from the UK and Ireland Confidential Enquiries into Maternal Deaths and Morbidity National Perinatal Epidemiology Unit. Oxford: University of Oxford; 2018.
3. Perlman M, Little H, Thompson B, Thompson R. Iconicity in signed and spoken vocabulary: a comparison between American sign language, British sign language, English, and Spanish. Front Psychol. 2018;9:37–51.
4. Murray J. Special issue: language planning and sign language rights. Sign Language Stud. 2015;15(4):375–8.
5. Action on Hearing Loss. Equal treatment? 2018.
6. Action on Hearing Loss. Good Practice? Wh"Action on Hearing Loss people who are deaf or have hearing loss still not getting accessible information from their GP; 2018.
7. Iqbal S. Pregnancy and birth: A guide for deaf Women. RNID and The National Childbirth Trust. London. 2004.
8. Evans L, Wu Y, Price E. A new hope? Experiences of accessibility of services in deaf and hard-of-hearing audiences post-digital television switchover. Int J Digit Telev. 2015;6(3):347–66.
9. Scullion PA. 'Disability' in a nursing curriculum. Disability Soc. 1999;14(4):539–59.
10. O'Hearn A. Deaf women's experiences and satisfaction with prenatal care: a comparative study. Medical care. 2006;12:p.13.
11. Wood H. The state of maternity care for women with disabilities. Women Birth. 2017;30:3.c.
12. Yoo G, Keum J, Hwang S, Ock YS. Development of the sign language translator system using Myo and RaspberryPi2. In: Proceedings of the annual conference of biomedical fuzzy systems association, vol 28, Biomedical Fuzzy Systems Association; 2015. p. 175–8.
13. Smeltzer SC, Mitra M, Long-Bellil L, Iezzoni LI, Smith LD. Obstetric clinicians' experiences and educational preparation for caring for pregnant women with physical disabilities: a qualitative study. Disabil Health J. 2018;11(1):8–13.
14. Smeijers AS, Pfau R. Towards a treatment for treatment: On communication between general practitioners and their deaf patients. The Sign Language Translator and Interpreter. 2009;3
15. Hoang L, LaHousse SF, Nakaji MC, Sadler GR. Assessing deaf cultural competency of physicians and medical students. J Cancer Educ. 2011;26(1):175–82.
16. Middleton A, Emery SD, Turner GH. Views, knowledge, and beliefs about genetics and genetic counseling among deaf people. Sign Lang Stud. 2010;10(2):170–96.
17. Tomlinson M, Swartz L, Officer A, Chan KY, Rudan I, Saxena S. Research priorities for health of people with disabilities: an expert opinion exercise. Lancet. 2009;374(9704):1857–62.
18. World Health Organisation (WHO). https://www.who.int/news-room/fact-sheets/detail/deafness-and-hearing-loss.
19. Jackson CW. Family supports and resources for parents of children who are deaf or hard of hearing. Am Ann Deaf. 2011;156(4):343–62.
20. Dedhia K, Graham E, Park A. Hearing loss and failed newborn hearing screen. Clin Perinatol. 2018;45(4):629–43.
21. Ledford CJW, Canzona MR, Womack JJ, Hodge JA. Influence of provider communication on women's delivery expectations and birth experience appraisal. Fam Med. 2016;48(7):523–31.
22. Schiff MA, Doody DR, Crane DA, Mueller BA. Pregnancy outcomes among deaf women in Washington State, 1987–2012. Obstet Gynecol. 2017;130(5):953.
23. Malouf R, Henderson J, Redshaw M. Access and quality of maternity care for disabled women during pregnancy, birth and the postnatal period in England: data from a national survey. BMJ Open. 2017;7(7):e016757.
24. McNally L. Existential sentences crosslinguistically: variations in form and meaning. Ann Rev Linguist. 2016;2:211–31.
25. Hubbard LJ, D'Andrea E, Carman LA. Promoting best practice for perinatal care of Deaf women. Nurs Womens Health. 2018;22(2):126–36.
26. Hodnett ED, Downe S, Walsh D. Alternative versus conventional institutional settings for birth. Cochrane Database Syst Rev. 2012;8

Breastfeeding Support for Women with Complex Social Needs

12

Abbi Ayers

Abstract

Breastfeeding support for women with complex social needs requires a proactive approach to understanding the barriers, triggers and inequalities they face when considering their infant feeding options and a proactive response to offering trauma-informed support that acknowledges and accounts for the multiple disadvantage, lived experience and deep-rooted trauma these women may bear. This chapter seeks to explore the key considerations health professionals, carers, policymakers and commissioners must take into account to achieve this. Furthermore, current evidence-based research and good practice clearly demonstrate that when women with complex social needs can access specialised breastfeeding support, the associated health and wellbeing outcomes are twofold. The improved maternal, neonatal and long-term health and wellbeing benefits are widely recognised and undisputed. However, the lesser understood and documented value that the breastfeeding experience holds for a mother recovering from trauma, abuse, poor mental health and multiple disadvantage is, at best, woefully underestimated and, at worst, completely undermined by standard practice. Breastfeeding offers health, hope and healing to women with complex social needs, so improving breastfeeding support for these mothers is a matter of paramount importance from an ethical, equitable and social perspective.

Keywords

Breastfeeding · Support · Infant feeding · Trauma informed

A. Ayers (✉)
Birth Companions, London, UK
e-mail: abbi@teamsandham.com

© Springer Nature Switzerland AG 2021
L. Abbott (ed.), *Complex Social Issues and the Perinatal Woman*,
https://doi.org/10.1007/978-3-030-58085-8_12

Breastfeeding support can be an ambiguous definition, prone to interpretation on a number of levels. For example, direct breastfeeding support may entail intensive one-to-one contact between a caregiver and a postnatal mother, whereas indirect breastfeeding support might include fostering a positive breastfeeding culture or facilitating regular opportunities for expectant mothers to ask questions and access information about their infant feeding choices. For the most part, all women need some form of direct and indirect breastfeeding support if they are to be able to successfully initiate and establish breastfeeding.

So when devising a model and means to offer breastfeeding support to women with complex social needs, there are a number of important questions to first consider. How might this woman feel about breastfeeding, and why might she feel that way? What obstacles will this woman need to overcome before she can start breastfeeding? How might specific barriers to breastfeeding impact a woman's physical and psychological ability to breastfeed? What approach will help ensure that this woman feels safe, listened to and understood? And how can we help instil and encourage this woman's confidence and sense of self-worth to best ensure that she and her baby benefit from their shared breastfeeding experience? The opportunity to breastfeed is afforded to every new mother who gives birth to a healthy baby. So follows, opportunities for us as health professionals and caregivers to offer both direct and indirect breastfeeding support to these mothers are plentiful and ongoing. However, when offering breastfeeding support to women with complex social needs, we need to take a step back from conventional and generic support models to be able to consider things from a different perspective. These women not only need evidence-based information and practical support with breastfeeding; they also need trauma-informed care, specialist advice and guidance and non-judgmental acceptance and empathy as they make the infant feeding choices that are right for them.

12.1 Main Barriers to Breastfeeding for Women with Complex Social Needs

In a society that instils the importance of convenience over sustenance and body consciousness over body function, it is hardly surprising that the UK has some of the worst breastfeeding initiation and prevalence rates in the world. We are not only missing countless opportunities to encourage and support women who want to breastfeed, but we are also failing them by enabling multiple barriers to breastfeeding to overshadow any concerted and meaningful efforts to normalise it. The average expectant mother will need to de-sensitize herself to a barrage of negative ideas and opinions about breastfeeding, wade through overwhelming amounts of inaccurate and inconsistent information about infant feeding choices, resist aggressive influencing and marketing techniques from formula milk manufacturers and proactively seek out reliable and credible support. And for women with complex social needs, the brick wall to breastfeeding has even stronger foundations deep-rooted in their past experiences, health inequalities and current life circumstances.

12.1.1 Perinatal Triggers

A compelling and rapidly developing body of evidence clearly demonstrates how experiences during pregnancy, labour, birth and breastfeeding have the potential to trigger past trauma for survivors of sexual violence and abuse [1–3]. Reactions to such triggers manifest themselves in a number of different ways. Survivors may experience flashbacks and/or emotional distress including depression, intrusion, anxiety or anger. Some may have difficulty developing and maintaining interpersonal relationships and may experience avoidance symptoms like disassociation or amnesia. Some may suffer from post-traumatic stress disorder (PTSD) or complex post-traumatic stress disorder (CPTSD). Survivors may experience cognitive distortions of their perceived reality or develop an impaired sense of self. And some may suffer from physical complaints and poor health such as fatigue, chronic pain, insomnia, infections and frequent headaches. Breastfeeding can play a significant role in re-traumatizing women who have experienced sexual violence and can often be presumed to be an unlikely infant feeding choice for survivors of sexual abuse.

12.1.2 Specific Breastfeeding Triggers

Exposing and sharing their body with another person can require immense strength and tenacity from the survivor, and having frequent and dependent physical contact with their baby can be re-traumatising in itself. It is also important to note that while some mothers initially feel comfortable breastfeeding their infant child, they may later struggle to breastfeed an older baby who is more playful and socially engaged at the breast. Older babies may naturally want to touch and fondle the breast as they suckle which can be a trigger to past trauma. Additionally, women who self-harm or bear the scars of self-harm or previous abuse may find it particularly difficult to reveal otherwise concealed parts of their body. These are unique barriers to breastfeeding that need to be widely recognised and sensitively addressed by any professional or caregiver involved in offering breastfeeding support. It is also very important to avoid making the assumption that survivors of abuse will not want to breastfeed. Many make a very deliberate and conscious decision to nurse their babies themselves, and with the right support, the act of breastfeeding can be hugely healing and therapeutic.

12.1.3 Medications and Breastfeeding

For women with complex mental health issues reliant on medication to treat conditions like anxiety, depression and panic attacks, breastfeeding can often be considered incompatible with their medicinal needs. Furthermore, a woman's decision and ability to breastfeed her baby may be compromised by conflicting information and recommendations from health professionals and caregivers. Being confused or overwhelmed by the information offered can make it impossible for women to ascertain whether or not breastfeeding is appropriate and safe for their babies. So it is important to understand and advocate the number of ways nursing mothers can use medication alongside safe breastfeeding practices. Furthermore, mounting evidence about the long-term mental health benefits to women who breastfeed adds weight to the argument that those suffering from or at risk of developing mental health issues should be supported to breastfeed as exhaustively as possible.

12.1.4 Demographics, Social Inequalities and Cultural Trends

Demographics dictate that women with complex social needs suffer from much higher rates of poverty, illiteracy, unemployment, poor health and diminished life chances [4–6]. These women are far less likely to enter further and higher education, more likely to need to overcome language barriers and communication issues and frequently foster a deep-rooted mistrust of statutory services and institutional support. These demographic factors leave women with complex social needs at a distinct disadvantage before breastfeeding can even be considered as a feeding choice. Inter-generational norms and familial expectations can also influence whether or not a woman chooses to breastfeed. Those with fragmented and displaced support networks and complicated interpersonal relationships often lack exposure to and involvement in a positive breastfeeding culture. They may never have seen a baby being breastfed before or talked to a mother who has enjoyed a positive breastfeeding experience. Additionally, for women in prison, social segregation and isolation have a further negative impact on a mother's opportunities to benefit from the shared life experiences, ongoing encouragement and peer support and advice from trusted sources with regard to their breastfeeding choices.

Furthermore, a bottle-feeding culture has become normalised and is now prevalent in our society [7, 8]. Aggressive formula milk marketing practices are poorly regulated due to the UK's non-compliance with the World Health Organization's (WHO) International Code of Marketing of Breastmilk Substitutes. There is also a distinct lack of positive breastfeeding role models in the mainstream media, and the emergence and popularity of multiple social media platforms put further pressure on women to conform to the norm. Women living in isolation or with very limited positive encouragement and influence from family, friends and a trusted support network will need to debunk social, cultural and demographic trends if they plan to breastfeed.

12.1.5 Mothers at Risk of Separation

Many women with complex social needs will be at risk of temporary, partial or permanent separation from their babies [9]. Some mothers will know to expect to separate from their babies after birth, and for these women, this knowledge will inform their infant feeding choices in advance. They may not want to consider breastfeeding in any capacity for fear of establishing a bond or connection with their baby that then makes separation all the more painful and traumatic. Or they might judge short-term breastfeeding to be pointless and may struggle to recognise the value of any breastfeeding over no breastfeeding at all. Other mothers might have to separate from their children unexpectedly or without preparation at a point after which breastfeeding has already been established. For these women, maintaining milk production by expressing, with a view to sharing their milk with their baby by other indirect means, can simply be a challenge too great to contemplate. Furthermore, the emotional distress and stress hormones can impair the physiology of lactation in the separated mother, making it more difficult for her to produce and collect her milk even if she wants to do so. Additionally, the physical discomfort and impact on postnatal recovery that a sudden cessation of breastfeeding can have on a woman's body can further inhibit breastfeeding to such an extent that breastfeeding is no longer physically possible.

Despite this veritable obstacle course of challenges, many women with complex social needs will remain determined and committed to breastfeeding. To nurture and nurse a newborn can give women an enormous sense of purpose, achievement and pride. Breastfeeding can open doors to deep and meaningful relationships for women who have otherwise struggled to find acceptance and love in their family units and social networks. And the very act of breastfeeding itself can help heal emotional and psychological scars from a lifetime of neglect, abuse, vulnerability and disadvantage.

The evidence attesting to the health, social and environmental benefits of breastfeeding is overwhelmingly compelling, but as health professionals, lactation consultants and support agencies working collaboratively to support women with complex social needs, it is our collective responsibility to challenge and dispel assumptions about the infant feeding choices these mothers may make. Along the way, we also need to recognise that these women need bespoke, trauma-informed, easily accessible and non-judgmental support to inform and empower them to breastfeed if they choose to do so.

12.2 Defining an Approach to Breastfeeding Support

It is important to consider all of these barriers to breastfeeding when defining an approach and model of breastfeeding support best suited and most effective for women with complex social needs.

Every expectant and new mother needs to be listened to with empathy and respect. And for those contemplating their infant feeding choices during pregnancy or those beginning their breastfeeding experience as new mothers, the opportunity to ask questions, debrief anxieties and offload emotions can be hugely helpful. As professionals, our duty of care includes offering current, evidence-based information and unbiased, non-judgmental support. With these principles inherent in any approach to breastfeeding support, we then also need to encompass a trauma-informed perspective and a willingness to seek out and offer bespoke and specialist information when supporting women with complex social needs.

12.2.1 Trauma-Informed Breastfeeding Support

Trauma-informed[1] breastfeeding support would presume that all women may have experienced or may currently be experiencing some form of trauma that might influence their infant feeding choices and compromise their natural ability to initiate and maintain breastfeeding. At this point, it is important to clarify that we should not assume the impact of this trauma will always be a negative one, and I will expand on this point later. Furthermore, adopting a trauma-informed approach to breastfeeding support need not be daunting or overly complicated for health professionals and caregivers. If a clear grasp of the key principles of trauma-informed care remains at the centre of all our work with women with complex social needs, a trauma-informed model of breastfeeding support will evolve naturally.

According to the Substance Abuse and Mental Health Services Administration (SAMHSA[2]), a trauma-informed approach needs to include the following:

- Realisation that trauma can have a widespread impact
- Recognition of the signs and symptoms of trauma in clients
- Responsiveness to a client's needs by integrating knowledge and understanding about trauma into any support offered
- A determined and active effort to resist re-traumatising the client

In terms of breastfeeding support for women with complex social needs, this means that we should assume all mothers have experienced trauma at some point in their lives, and this assumption should inform and influence the way we offer information, encouragement and guidance around infant feeding choices.

12.2.2 Supporting Survivors of Sexual Abuse

When it comes to offering breastfeeding support for a mother who has or may still be experiencing sexual abuse, we must first remind ourselves of our remit. It is not our role to encourage women to debrief and address these experiences or offer counsel, diagnosis or intervention (although safeguarding concerns should always be escalated as part of our professional duty of care). Also, recognising and understanding some of the main reasons why a survivor of sexual abuse may not want to breastfeed or struggle to do so is crucial. With very little meaningful research into the effects of sexual abuse on breastfeeding, many of the conclusions we can draw are based on empirical and anecdotal evidence, and it is this evidence base we must use to inform our approach and practice.

Many survivors of sexual abuse experience discomfort, anxiety and distress when they are in a situation that replicates feelings of exposure, exploitation and

---

[1] See Chap. 13.
[2] Substance Abuse and Mental Health Services Administration (SAMHSA).

vulnerability. So as caregivers, it is important that we recognise and acknowledge that breastfeeding can be such a situation.

The long-term effects of sexual abuse can also affect a woman's functioning and reasoning, coping strategies, stress management skills and general health and well-being [1]. Survivors may develop a very negative and disparaging sense of self. They may suffer from low self-esteem and might underestimate their ability to care for and feed their babies themselves. If survivors can overcome these feelings of inadequacy to the point they initiate breastfeeding, a perceived lack of self-efficacy might make it difficult or even impossible for them to ask for support. And if their initial breastfeeding efforts are unsuccessful, survivors may attribute this to their own personal failings.

So with these many considerations in mind, many women will simply not contemplate breastfeeding or persist with breastfeeding. Even with good intent and an evidence base behind us, questioning a woman's decision not to breastfeed or to stop breastfeeding, or trying to persuade her to persist, not only might undermine a woman's confidence and self-esteem but could have a negative impact on her long-term emotional wellbeing and mental health. As care providers, we therefore need to continually remind ourselves of these complexities and sensitivities to enable us to facilitate and deliver an appropriate and woman-centred level of breastfeeding support.

12.2.3 Survivors Who Breastfeed

Many survivors of sexual abuse do however make the very deliberate and empowering decision to breastfeed, and their motivation may actually be rooted in their trauma history. Through my work with Birth Companions, I have frequently supported survivors of CSA who have made the deeply committed decision to take back ownership of their bodies and embrace their unique ability to offer their child their milk. This opportunity can feel daunting, frightening even, but it can also be hugely empowering to a woman who has previously lost her personal autonomy. These women talk about the pride and empowerment they experience by being able to breastfeed their babies. Some are first-time mothers, whereas others may have exclusively bottle-fed their older children but, with support, choose to breastfeed at a time in their lives when they feel strong enough to do so.

Whereas previously a woman might have struggled with feelings of shame, humiliation, pain or disgust with regard to her body, breastfeeding can help redefine that relationship. She can offer breastmilk to her baby, as only a mother can; she can feel awe at her physical ability to nurture and sustain another human being with the milk her body produces; and she can enjoy the closeness and bonding that breastfeeding facilitates. When we are able to offer breastfeeding support in these instances, simply helping mothers to acknowledge and celebrate their capacity for breastfeeding can be hugely impactful. And through my work with survivors of CSA, I have seen first-hand that when a woman has the opportunity and support to make the decision to breastfeed, even for just one feed, she can regain control of her choices, take pride and pleasure in her body and begin a process of self-healing and self-nurture.

Case Study

Selina was pregnant with her third child when we first met her at a Birth Companions' pregnancy group session. She did not have custody of her older children who both lived with her extended family, but Selina had regular contact with them. She was experiencing reoccurring trauma and anxiety as a result of her separation from her children.

Selina had multiple complex social needs including a history of childhood abuse, being a LAC, Social Services involvement, substance misuse and poor mental health. She had never breastfeed before and had assumed that bottle feeding was her only option, particularly as she was preparing to separate from her baby shortly after giving birth.

We spent time talking to Selina about her options around infant feeding, both as part of a general group discussion and on a one-to-one basis. Through this support contact, we observed how Selina began to consider breastfeeding as a positive step to beginning to reshape her relationship with her body and to facilitating bonding between herself and her baby before separation. She became increasingly committed to breastfeeding as her pregnancy progressed, and after giving birth, Selina was supported to offer baby Matthew his first colostrum feeds in hospital.

Matthew was discharged to the care of his paternal grandmother and Selina continued to access postnatal support from Birth Companions on a one-to-one basis for a number of weeks. She remained determined to express and collect her breastmilk to be stored and later transported to Matthew, and she received ongoing practical support to do this. Providing her milk for her son in this way helped Selina to achieve a sense of responsibility and self-worth in her role as a mother.

> *... although I have two other children I didn't breastfeed ... the right amount of advice and support encouraged me to try, which I loved. My son could benefit which is the best thing I ever did.—Selina*

Selina's story highlights how survivors of CSA can feel motivated and empowered to breastfeed in the most challenging of circumstances.

For those mothers who experience complicated and conflicting emotions and triggers to past trauma while breastfeeding, we can help them better identify when and why they may feel most vulnerable—physically, emotionally and psychologically—with a view to developing self-help and coping strategies. For example, a woman who was regularly abused as a child in her bedroom at night-time may find the night feeds particularly difficult. To address this, she may feel more comfortable if she gets out of bed, puts the lights on and breastfeeds in an arm chair. Or she may have the option of delegating night feeds to someone else, enabling her to avoid a possible routine of re-triggering behaviour. For survivors experiencing flashbacks or feelings of numbing or disassociation, it may help to play music or use potent scents and essential oils to create an environment that helps women to remain present and grounded. Some mothers may be confused or conflicted about the sensory pleasure that can be derived from breastfeeding. Explaining that this is completely normal and appropriate may help reassure a woman who might otherwise be struggling to rationalize the thoughts and feelings she experiences while breastfeeding.

Mothers who find it difficult to breastfeed as their baby gets older and more play-ful on the breast may benefit from better understanding their child's developmental norms. Touching, stroking and squeezing the breast during feeds are typical social and physiological behaviours for the older baby and can also assist in increasing and regulating the flow of breastmilk and promote bonding and oxytocin production crucial to the mechanics of breastfeeding itself. By offering a mother an alternative interpretation of her baby's behaviour at the breast, it may help her to better manage any complicated emotions she experiences while breastfeeding.

In addition to the psychological and emotional triggers that can affect the breast-feeding experience for survivors of sexual abuse, women's general physical health can also be negatively affected by their adverse childhood experiences [10] and past trauma. Mothers suffering from poor general health are at a greater risk of develop-ing blocked milk ducts, slower let down and milk transfer, mastitis and fatigue. Highlighting the importance of eating, drinking and sleeping regularly, alongside tailored self-care techniques like breast massage for engorgement or alternative positions to increase milk transfer, may help to better equip women to overcome the physical demands of breastfeeding.

But when mothers are being re-traumatised by their breastfeeding experience to the extent that they choose to avoid or stop breastfeeding altogether, demonstrating understanding and sensitivity is paramount. Survivors of sexual abuse may not attri-bute their decision to stop breastfeeding to their trauma history, and it is not our job to make the link for them. To maintain a trauma-informed approach to breastfeeding support, we must remind ourselves to avoid problem-solving and offering advice and to instead empower survivors with a voice and choice.

12.2.4 Breastfeeding Alongside Treatment for Mental Health Issues

Alongside the need for us to adopt a trauma-informed approach to breastfeeding support for women with complex social needs, we must also recognise when these women need specialist breastfeeding information that falls outside of our skill set and knowledge base. For example, for those taking medication for mental health issues, those combating addiction or substance misuse or those with specific health issues like HIV or hep B, we have a responsibility to provide credible information and make appropriate referrals to inform and empower a mother to make the infant feeding choice best suited to her situation.

Women with complex social needs have an increased risk of suffering from mental health issues and are thereby more likely to require medicinal treatment. Antidepressants can often be considered incompatible with breastfeeding by prescribing health professionals, and this is another example of when assumptive and blanket recommendations can be detrimental to health outcomes. The NHS guidelines state "the use of antidepressants if you're breastfeeding isn't usually recommended. However there are circumstances when both the benefits of treatment for depression (or other mental health conditions) and the benefits of breastfeeding your baby outweigh the potential risks [11]". So with this in mind, it can be helpful to have a basic understanding of variables that contribute to a medication's suitability for use by a nursing mother.

Drugs that are highly bound by maternal proteins are unable to diffuse in significant amounts into breastmilk and drugs with a low plasma: milk ratio reach the breastmilk in much smaller quantities. Additionally, medications with a short half-life are prevented from accumulating in a baby's system in potent amounts for extended periods [12, 13]. The quantity of breast milk that a baby receives will also influence how much medication they are exposed to as well as the age of the baby who is being breastfed; newborns ingest more milk and have more immature digestive systems than 6-month-old babies who have begun to wean. So a mother who is dependent on medication or drug replacement therapy (DRT) for her own wellbeing will need to be supported by professionals who have a full and detailed understanding of her medical needs and options and who can recognise when to refer her to specialist advisory services like the Breastfeeding Network's Drugs in Breastmilk information service [14]. It is also important to point to the emerging body of evidence that links breastfeeding with a reduced risk of developing postnatal depression (PND). A number of studies, including a recent large-scale study published by the University of Cambridge in 2014 [15], have demonstrated the link between positive breastfeeding experiences and improved maternal mental health outcomes. Breastfeeding facilitates enhanced interactions between mother and baby and increases positive physical, social and psychological responsiveness. Mothers who breastfeed have more opportunities to facilitate physical contact with their babies (skin to skin, eye contact, stroking), and the physiology of breastfeeding necessitates the regular production of feel-good hormones like oxytocin, naturally reducing stress responses. However, breastfeeding difficulties can contribute to increased levels of stress, anxiety and depression, demonstrating once again why trauma-informed and bespoke breastfeeding support is crucial for women with complex social needs.

12.2.5 Supporting Addicted Mothers

Women who are opioid dependent and on drug rehabilitation programs may also be told that breastfeeding is not safe for their babies, and as with antidepressants, there are variables to consider here too[3]. Research into maternal use of methadone demonstrates that breastfeeding has clear benefits for infants who have been exposed to the drug in utero [16–20]. Methadone enters breastmilk in very low quantities and concentrations, but when these small doses are ingested by the breastfed baby, withdrawal symptoms in addicted infants can be reduced or even eradicated. Babies born to opioid-dependent mothers are at greater risk of developing neonatal abstinence syndrome (NAS), but the available research also shows that when these babies are breastfed for the first 3 days (or more) after birth, they are significantly less likely to require treatment for NAS. In addition to the way small quantities of the drug in the milk lessen withdrawal symptoms, the combined health benefits of the breastmilk itself along with the way breastfeeding can soothe and calm an agitated infant have an overall positive impact on the baby's health outcomes.

When offering breastfeeding support to women with complex social needs, it is also important to recognise that this group of mothers is at a higher risk of developing poor lifestyle habits including smoking and frequent alcohol use. Some women may consider smoking as a barrier to breastfeeding, so it can be helpful to highlight the additional benefits of breastfeeding for the baby of a mother who smokes, including enhanced protection from respiratory issues and illness associated with exposure to secondary cigarette smoke [21, 22]. We can also discuss safer smoking practices for breastfeeding mothers to adopt such as only smoking after a feed so as to avoid peak levels of nicotine entering the breastmilk. Some mothers may also worry about the quantity of alcohol that passes into their milk. So offering information about safe breastfeeding practices for these mothers is invaluable. As caregivers, we are also in a position to instigate discussions around co-sleeping safety with an objective to ensure that women understand the associated risks of co-sleeping after smoking and alcohol use and are fully informed of the guidelines.

12.2.6 Breastfeeding with Infectious Diseases

Women with complex social needs are more likely to suffer from a number of specific health issues that are often considered to be prohibitive to breastfeeding, specifically in developed countries where there is good access to modern medicine, healthcare and clean water. These include hepatitis B or HIV[4]. The WHO [23] and UNICEF recommend that all infants be exclusively breastfed up to 6 months of age and that they continue to breastfeed up to 2 years of age or beyond with the addition of adequate complementary foods from about 6 months. This includes infants of mothers with the hep B and HIV virus.

With specific regard to Hep B, the WHO [24] states that there is no evidence that mothers who are chronic hepatitis B (HBV) carriers pose an additional risk of infecting their babies with HBV, despite small quantities of hepatitis B surface antigen (HBsAg) being detectable in some breastmilk samples. Furthermore, although

---

[3] See Chap. 3.
[4] See Chap. 8.

the WHO also recommends that all infants should receive the Hep B vaccine as part of their routine childhood immunization program, they also note that there is no enhanced risk for breastfed infants of mothers with Hep B without immunization, and any risk of transmission of the virus through breastmilk itself is entirely negligible compared to the much higher risk of exposure to maternal blood and bodily fluids at birth.

Similarly, the WHO recommends that HIV-positive mothers can safely breastfeed their babies with minimal risk of transferal of the virus via breastmilk and should be supported to do so. To facilitate this, the WHO also recommends that exclusive breastfeeding should be encouraged for the first 6 months before introducing appropriate complementary food and continuing to breastfeed up to 12 months. The WHO also advises that HIV-positive mothers take antiretroviral drugs before initiating breastfeeding and while continuing breastfeeding up until their babies are 12 months old.

In the UK, the British HIV Association (BHIVA) recommends [25] that the safest way for a mother with HIV to feed her baby is with formula milk since this negates any risk of HIV transmission after birth. However, the BHIVA guidelines recognise that mothers with HIV can be supported to breastfeed safely if a mother's viral load is undetectable and both mother and child undertake antiretroviral therapy (ART) and are healthy and free from infection, and mothers can be continually supported while breastfeeding so as to avoid any injury or damage to their breasts that could lead to cracks, inflammation or mastitis that carry an increased risk of HIV transmission.

With all this in mind, offering non-judgmental support and encouraging informed choice are once again the linchpins of good breastfeeding support. For women dealing with the physical challenges, emotional distress and social stigma associated with being a carrier of an infectious disease, the value of a trauma-informed approach to breastfeeding support is further underlined. These women may not be susceptible to trauma triggers per say, but they too might find the physical act of breastfeeding to be very stressful and may be further challenged by negative self-perception and self-esteem issues and general poor health.

12.2.7 Delivering Support That Remains Sensitive to the Individual

In addition to these very specific physical, psychological and mental health issues that women with complex social needs may be dealing with alongside breastfeeding, some may also need to overcome the social, cultural and practical challenges to breastfeeding that are associated with their current circumstances and life situation. Women within this demographic group frequently lead very chaotic lifestyles that can make it difficult for them to access regular support and reliable information. They may lack the social and communication skills needed to articulate and express their needs and might struggle to be proactive in asking for help. Social inequalities could make it more difficult for these mothers to successfully engage with drop-in groups and peer support, and high levels of mistrust in statutory services may lead to women feeling reluctant or unwilling to disclose their concerns or anxieties to health professionals and caregivers for fear of unwanted repercussions and intervention. Furthermore, some of these women may be at risk of detention, may have recently been released from custody or may be serving time in prison during their perinatal period. For these women, breastfeeding and parenting choices may feel very limited, and access to ongoing and consistent support will likely be compromised.

With all of this in mind, breastfeeding support for these women needs to be unconditional, non-judgmental and entirely flexible. Recognising when one-to-one support will be more effectual than group support and vice versa, understanding why women may remain elusive or might be difficult or reluctant to engage, demonstrating sensitivity and empathy when women make irrational or irresponsible decisions around feeding practices and early parenting choices, adopting core counselling skills to best establish how a woman feels about her feeding options and offering information on the basis of what she needs to know not what we think she should know—these are all characteristics of good breastfeeding support for women's complex social needs.

12.3 Recognising the Value and Benefits of Offering Breastfeeding Support to Women with Complex Social Needs

12.3.1 What Breastfeeding Prevalence Rates Can Tell Us

All breastfeeding support is designed to increase positive breastfeeding outcomes including and perhaps most highly valued, improved short- and long-term health benefits for mothers and babies. Breastfeeding initiation rates offer us an insight into how effective and influential positive breastfeeding messages and information have been on pregnant women who elect to initiate breastfeeding immediately after giving birth. But it is breastfeeding prevalence rates—the percentage of women still breastfeeding in some capacity at 6–8 weeks postnatally—that give us a clearer indication of how impactful breastfeeding support can be. Since the discontinuation of the National Infant Feeding Survey in 2010, breastfeeding initiation and prevalence rates have been collected and collated by individual local authorities with specific key performance indicators being monitored and reported on. With this in mind, it is necessary to note that because local authorities are required to pass three levels of validation in order for their statistics to be included, and because data collection methods can be inconsistent or incomprehensive, there has been a decline in data quality since the last Infant Feeding Survey in 2010. That said, the most recent statistics available [26] demonstrate a clear and urgent need for improvements to breastfeeding support for all women in the UK with less than half (43%) of mothers in England still breastfeeding their babies in some capacity 6–8 weeks after birth.

As UNICEF points out, an increase in breastfeeding rates would directly and dramatically improve child health; reduce incidences of childhood illnesses such as ear, chest and gut infections; and potentially save the NHS up to £50 million each year. UNICEF also asserts that "a key aspect of improving breastfeeding rates is the provision of face-to-face, ongoing, predictable support for families across all public services and social support in the community" [27]. The UNICEF Baby Friendly Initiative aims to facilitate this by raising standards for breastfeeding support across perinatal services.

So there is clear-cut evidence for why breastfeeding support directly improves health and wellbeing outcomes for mothers and babies as well as indirectly benefitting public services, the NHS and society in general. However, in addition to these generic benefits, there are further positive outcomes derived from supporting women with complex social needs to breastfeed that can sometimes be overlooked or undervalued.

12.3.2 The Benefits of Breastfeeding Support for Women with Complex Social Needs

Working closely with these new mothers affords us opportunities to acknowledge, address and better understand negative or reluctant feelings around breastfeeding and other early parenting choices. We are also well placed to offer credible, evidence-based information to enable women to make educated and informed decisions for themselves. In doing so, these women can subsequently experience improved confidence and competence levels and increased self-esteem. Being able to successfully establish breastfeeding can often lead women to make positive changes across all aspects of their lifestyle. They may begin to take better care of themselves physically by developing consistent daily routines and improving their diet. They may be more motivated to address addictive behaviours such as a dependence on alcohol or smoking to relieve stress. Furthermore, for these women, an emotional investment in another human being may increase feelings of self-worth, self-respect, dignity and a heightened sense of responsibility.

The very act of accessing breastfeeding support can facilitate a regular and ongoing contact between new mothers and their health professionals. In turn, this may help women develop trust and a renewed faith in statutory services. In some instances, women may even develop positive supportive relationships with individual caregivers which can have a long-lasting impact on their willingness to engage with and access support in the future.

Opportunities to receive non-judgmental, unconditional and consistent support can also contrast dramatically with the chaos and instability of other aspects of their lifestyle. For example, for women trapped in troubled relationships or embroiled in difficult legal or financial situations, the continuity of support and the empathy demonstrated by their caregivers can be very welcoming and reassuring at a time when they may feel particularly vulnerable and alone.

If women are receptive to accessing group support, the social links and networks that breastfeeding drop-in groups or support services offer new mums can prove invaluable for the long-term health and wellbeing of the family unit. Group and peer support can help increase women's confidence and willingness to socialise. New mothers attending breastfeeding support groups can develop closer links with other groups and services in their community, helping to reduce their isolation and enabling them to benefit from other positive influences and the shared experiences of other new mums.

The impact of breastfeeding support for women with complex social needs is twofold and can perhaps be best categorised in primary (generic) outcomes and secondary (bespoke) outcomes. All mothers who breastfeed and all babies who are breastfed will benefit from the well-documented and substantiated short- and long-term health and wellbeing outcomes we know so well. But women with complex social needs are also likely to benefit from a secondary tier of outcomes that relate specifically to their personal circumstances and vulnerabilities including opportunities to re-evaluate and redefine the way they feel about their bodies; an improved sense of self-respect and self-worth; feelings of achievement and empowerment; improved relationships with their health professionals and wider support networks; and a chance to nurture and bond with their babies in ways that can help heal and repair the turbulence and trauma of their life experiences.

12.3.3 Breastfeeding Support for Women with Complex Social Needs

Breastfeeding support for women with complex social needs is in itself complex. It firstly requires us to develop a comprehensive and detailed understanding of the many barriers to breastfeeding that this particular group of women need to address and overcome. We must then approach breastfeeding support from a trauma-informed perspective with a remit to offering women trauma-informed care and support both during their pregnancies as they begin to consider their infant feeding choices and postnatally as they adapt to the realities of motherhood and the demands of breastfeeding alongside the challenges of their personal circumstances. Thereafter, we have a responsibility to tailor support to the appropriate level, offer evidence-based and credible information as required, refer to specialist support as needed and avoid making assumptive and blanket recommendations outside of our remit. Finally, it helps to remind ourselves that aside from the health and wellbeing benefits that breastfeeding affords mother and babies, there are a number of additional and often undervalued ways in which breastfeeding support benefits this group of women in social and interpersonal ways.

The opportunity for a mother to breastfeed her baby in any capacity is one that health professionals and caregivers need to highly value and fiercely protect. All and any breastfeeding can have a positive impact and for women with complex social needs, and this impact can be all the more important for both the short- and long-term physical and mental health and wellbeing of the mother. Breastfeeding helps and breastfeeding heals, and breastfeeding support is pivotal in enabling women with complex social needs not only to embrace and value their responsibilities as caregivers but to also thrive in their roles as mothers.

References

1. Simkin P, Klaus P. When survivors give birth. Seattle, WA: Classic Day. Quality Code Publisher; 2004.
2. Kendall-Taskett K. Breastfeeding and the sexual abuse survivor. J Hum Lact. 1998;14:125–30. University of New Hampshire.
3. Taylor J, Seng J. Trauma-informed care for in the perinatal period. Dunedin: Academic Press; 2015.
4. Lindquist A, Kurinczuk JJ, Redshaw M, Knight M. Experiences, utilisation and outcomes of maternity care in England among women from different socio-economic groups: findings from the 2010 National Maternity Survey. Oxford, UK: National Perinatal Epidemiology Unit, Nuffield Department of Population Health, University of Oxford; 2017.
5. Marmot M, Allen J, Goldblatt P et al. Fair society, healthy lives: strategic review of health inequalities in England post 2010. Marmot Review Team; 2010.
6. McNeish D, Scott S. Women and girls at risk—evidence across the life course. Literature Review; 2014.
7. Brown A. Who really decides how we feed our babies. London: Pinter & Martin; 2016.
8. Palmer G. The politics of breastfeeding: when breasts are bad for business. London: Pinter & Martin; 2009.
9. Broadhurst K. Vulnerable birth mothers and recurrent care proceedings. Lancaster University; 2014–2018.
10. Felitti VJ, Anda RF, Nordenberg D et al. The Adverse Childhood Experiences Study: Relationship of childhood abuse and household dysfunction to many of the leading causes of death in adults. Elsevier Science Inc.; 1998.
11. NHS Guidelines on cautions of use of antidepressants during pregnancy and breastfeeding. Last updated August 2018.
12. Jones W. MRPharmS and the breastfeeding network: introduction to the safety of drugs passing through breastmilk; 2019 Sep.
13. Hotham N. Drugs in breastfeeding. Adelaide: University of South Australia; 2015.
14. https://www.breastfeedingnetwork.org.uk/detailed-information/drugs-in-breastmilk/
15. Borra C, Iacovou M, Sevilla A. New Evidence on breastfeeding and postpartum depression: the importance of understanding women's intentions. Matern Child Health. 2015;19:897–907.
16. Abdel-Latif ME, Pinner J, Clews S, Cooke F, et al. Effects of breastmilk on the severity and outcome of neonatal abstinence syndrome among infants of drug-dependent mothers. Am Acad Pediatrics. 2006;117:e1163–9.
17. Jansson LM. ABM Clinical Protocol #21: guidelines for breastfeeding and the drug-dependent woman. Breastfeed Med. 2009;4:225–8.
18. Jansson LM, Choo R, Velez ML, Harrow C, Schroeder JR, Shakleya DM, Huestis MA. Methadone maintenance and breastfeeding in the neonatal period. Pediatrics. 2008;121:869.
19. Sharpe C, Kuschel C. Outcomes of infants born to mothers receiving methadone for pain management in pregnancy. Arch Dis Child Fetal Neonatal Ed. 2004;89:F33–6.
20. Glatstein M, Garcia-Bournissen F, Finkelstein Y, Koren G. Methadone exposure during lactation. Can Fam Physician. 2008;54:1689–90.
21. NHS guidelines on breastfeeding and smoking; 2018 Dec.
22. La Leche League Great Britain. Guidelines on Smoking and breastfeeding; 2016.
23. The World Health Organization. Breastfeeding guidelines; 2020.

24. Global Programme for Vaccines and Immunization (GPV) and the Divisions of Child Health and Development (CHD), and Reproductive Health (Technical Support) (RHT) World Health Organization. Statement on Hepatitis B and breastfeeding; 1996.
25. British HIV Association Guidelines for the management of HIV infection in pregnant women; 2018.
26. Public Health England. Official statistics breastfeeding prevalence at 6-8 weeks after birth (experimental statistics) quarter 4 2017/18 statistical commentary; July 2018.
27. UNICEF United Kingdom—the baby friendly initiative: breastfeeding—a public health issue; 2019.

Birth Companions and How We Came to Work in a Trauma-Informed Way

13

Denise Marshall

Abstract

Birth Companions is a unique charity working with women facing challenges and extreme disadvantage in the perinatal period. At the end of 1995, a pregnant woman in Holloway prison wrote to the Association for Improvement in Maternity Services (AIMS) about her situation and was supported by Beverley Beech who filmed, with a concealed camera, the woman shackled and accompanied by prison officers while in labour. This footage was shown on television and shone a spotlight about this marginalised group of women in prison. After this, women were rarely shackled or handcuffed in labour, but many still gave birth alone. Birth campaigner Sheila Kitzinger organised a meeting, and from this, Birth Companions (originally the Holloway Doula Group) was formed. The volunteers who came together were antenatal teachers, midwives and doulas who understood that this was a crucial time in mothers and babies' lives. The group wanted to ensure that women from prison would have emotional and practical support while giving birth and that these mothers and babies would have the best start possible. Birth Companions volunteers draw on a long tradition of female family and community members supporting women around the time of birth. Birth Companions approach is warm and caring, and women often say that the birth companions are like friends or family. Volunteers are trained to support women in a way that is safe and professional, protecting the women and the volunteers. The style and philosophy of Birth Companions are rooted in the trauma-informed approach it has developed in response to the needs and past experiences of the women they support. The service has developed since its conception in 1996 where antenatal, birth and postpartum support for women who were pregnant in prison was first offered. Collaborative working, peer to peer support and women who are expert by experience in the Birth Companions lived expe-

D. Marshall (✉)
Head of Services, Birth Companions, London, UK
e-mail: denise@birthcompanions.org.uk

© Springer Nature Switzerland AG 2021
L. Abbott (ed.), *Complex Social Issues and the Perinatal Woman*,
https://doi.org/10.1007/978-3-030-58085-8_13

rience team have shaped the way in which the charity works with staff, volunteers and women. Birth Companions has come to understand that it can be systems and services, rather than the women, that can be "difficult to engage with".

Keywords

Birth companions · Trauma-informed approaches · Lived experience teams · Volunteering · Prisoners · Community link

13.1 Introduction

Birth Companions (Fig. 13.1) is a unique charity working with women facing challenges and disadvantage in the perinatal period. The organisation began in 1996 after publicity about a woman from Holloway Prison being shackled in labour [1]. Although the charity has grown and now works with women in the community in London, as well as working in four other prisons, the harsh environment of this early prison setting was a strong influence in shaping our ethos and way of working. More recently, we have become aware of the literature around working in a trauma-informed way and have realised that this very much describes our approach with women, as well as how we look after our staff and volunteers. This chapter will explore how the Birth Companions' way of working developed and what it means in practice. It will hopefully provide useful insights for others working with women with complex needs in the perinatal period, both in the statutory and voluntary sectors.

Fig. 13.1 Birth companions logo (https://www.birthcompanions.org.uk/)

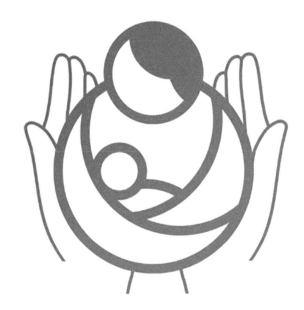

13.2   History and Early Influences

At the end of 1995, a pregnant woman in Holloway prison wrote to the Association for Improvement in Maternity Services (AIMS) about her situation, and Beverley Beech, from AIMS, agreed to be her birth partner [2]. While supporting her, Beverley filmed, with a concealed camera, Anette shackled and accompanied by prison officers while in labour. This footage was shown on television and shone a spotlight on the situation of this hidden and marginalised group of women in prison. After this, women were rarely shackled or handcuffed in labour, but many still gave birth alone. Birth writer and campaigner Sheila Kitzinger organised a meeting, and from this, Birth Companions (originally the Holloway Doula Group) was formed. The volunteers who came together were antenatal teachers, midwives and doulas who understood that this was a crucial time in mothers and babies' lives. The group wanted to ensure that women from the prison would have emotional and practical support while giving birth and that these mothers and babies would have the best start possible.

The prison, reeling with the bad publicity, agreed that Birth Companions could support women when they went out to give birth at the Whittington Hospital. They also allowed the birth companions into Holloway to meet the pregnant women in an antenatal class which was part of the prison's Education Department. I had just started as the antenatal teacher and worked closely with Birth Companions to ensure that the volunteers could visit weekly to meet pregnant women and offer them birth support. The women welcomed the opportunity to have this one-to-one time with a birth companion, to do a birth plan or to talk about whatever was on their mind. Many women said that it helped them to feel less anxious knowing that they could have a birth companion. As one woman put it "I felt safer knowing that I would not be alone for the birth". The classes could be busy, and sometimes officers or others would need to interrupt, but, despite this, we managed to create a feeling of normality and safety, where women could focus on their pregnancy and developing baby. Outside of the group, the prison could be a harsh environment. Women described feeling fearful for their safety. Some worried about being targeted or accidentally being caught up in a fight, but the biggest fear was not being unlocked in time when they went into labour or had a medical emergency. The birth companions reacted instinctively: they realised that they needed to build trust with the women and to offer reassurance and find ways to reduce the high levels of anxiety that they encountered.

The doula approach of trying to make the environment for birth feel "safe" was exactly what was needed when women had prison officers with them in early labour and, sometimes, while actually giving birth. Doula is a Greek word meaning "to serve" and is used today to describe a lay woman who supports a mother in the perinatal period. This idea of "serving" or honouring the wishes of the woman was also important. Women, by virtue of being in prison, are hugely disempowered. The birth companions talked with women about their fears but also about their wishes, and the birth plan was a way to explore choices that women could make for their birth and time in hospital with their baby.

The Birth Companions volunteers were drawing on a long tradition of female family and community members supporting women around the time of birth. Adela Stockton, in her book *Gentle Birth Companions: Doulas Serving Humanity* (2010), described the modern doula movement in the UK as a response to the erosion of communities and hospitalisation of birth, which can leave mothers feeling isolated and uncared for at this important time [3]. Today, women in Britain are often giving birth away from family and without having support in their local community. This situation is even more extreme for women who are giving birth while in prison. Many women said that having the support from Birth Companions, particularly at the birth, made them feel like they had family around them. As one woman put it:

It made you feel good, less left out. They made up for what I was missing, my family. (Seiko)

Another aspect of the support was listening to women but not asking them about their offence or why they were in prison. This felt like the right thing to do so that it was clear that the birth companions were non-judgemental and there to support them as pregnant women, regardless of their history or why they were in prison. The women in the group told us how much they valued feeling like a pregnant woman or a new mum, not a prisoner. One woman wrote:

When I arrived at the group, I felt so welcome, reassured and, even more importantly, accepted. I was encouraged to speak, never asked about why I was in prison and felt comfortable enough to open up about my hopes, fears and expectations as a mother to be. For two hours it felt like we were a normal group of mums and I can honestly say you forget where you are. (Deja)

When midwives first came into prison from the Whittington Hospital in 1998, the women again said how much they appreciated being treated as a "normal pregnant woman [1]". Previously, antenatal care was delivered in-house, and sadly, some health professionals in prison had become institutionalised. There was a culture of disbelief when women reported feeling unwell or thought they were in labour. A common response was that women just wanted "a trip out to hospital", and one birth companion remembers being told by a prison nurse that a woman did "not deserve support". Birth Companions worked closely with the Whittington midwives in prison and at the hospital, and with Hibiscus [4], a charity providing language, legal and other support for women who are foreign nationals (over 20% of women in Holloway) [5]. Signposting and working in partnership are a strong feature of Birth Companions' work today, and this collaborative approach really benefits the women we work with. Although Holloway prison closed in 2016, Birth Companions has been working with perinatal women in Bronzefield and Peterborough prisons for several years. We are now starting groups in two other prisons, Foston Hall and Low Newton. These prisons hold pregnant women and women recently separated from a baby but do not have Mother and Baby Units. In this new project, we are working with Fiona Dry, a midwife who has been doing some pioneering work to recognise the continued perinatal and mental health needs of women in prison up to 1 year post-birth.

Penny Simkin, childbirth writer and trainer, was invited to do an early training for the birth companions on comfort measures in labour. Her works *The Birth Partner* (1989) [6] and, later, *When Survivors Give Birth* (2004) [7] were key reading. Simkin's later book [7] describes how the past trauma of survivors of childhood sexual abuse can be triggered around the perinatal period and how birth partners can support women in ways that help them not to be re-traumatised. Key to this is listening to the woman's wishes. The approach that Penny Simkin was advocating for supporting survivors of childhood sexual abuse felt very relevant to the needs of the women in Holloway; and many of her experiences supporting women resonated with those of the birth companions. Another influence was Sheila Kitzinger, who agreed to become the patron of Birth Companions and championed the charity's work. Sheila had also written about trauma and birth and brought this awareness to the group.

13.3 The Common Thread of Trauma

Although birth companions never asked women about their lives, it seemed that once women felt safe, they wanted to open up and tell their story. Either in the group or one to one or often while in early labour, women talked about their lives and how they had ended up in prison. Women talked about having their baby taken away shortly after giving birth. It felt like women needed to feel listened to and that perhaps no one had listened to them before. The stories were often experiences of trauma and could be harrowing. Women talked about being exploited and abused by a parent and then a partner or about how their life had "fallen apart" after a bereavement. Women described the trauma of having a baby removed from their care shortly after giving birth. Many women had experienced sexual violence, and sometimes this baby was the result of rape. This was sometimes the case for women who had been trafficked or were fleeing war situations. It was shocking that some women were only in prison because they had entered the country illegally while running away from family or state violence. For other women, their lives were so hard on the outside that prison felt like a place of safety for them. This was the case for women with violent partners or women struggling with substance misuse or for women living on the street. Some women visibly thrived while in prison because they had three meals a day and shelter and felt safer than when they were not in prison. Some women had just made a bad choice or had unwittingly been implicated in a crime, often by their partner.

For many women, coming into prison was, in itself, traumatic, especially if this meant being separated from children. Most women in prison are separated from a child who they were caring for before they came to prison, and most children's lives change dramatically. Children have to move home and school and sometimes go into foster care. As well as the pain and guilt of being separated from a baby or older child, women also feel high levels of stress about giving birth from prison and whether they will get a place on the prison Mother and Baby Unit. (See Abbott's chapter for more details about women in prison.) Trauma was a persistent thread, and there were many aspects of prison life that could be triggers for women's past experiences of trauma, including loss of control, authority figures, restraint and fear for their physical safety.

The perinatal period can be very challenging for women who have experienced trauma, with the physical and emotional changes of pregnancy, physical examinations, pain, lack of privacy and the demands of a new baby. The women in Holloway had many fears around giving birth but found coming to the group reassuring. They liked that we were there every week and that when we said that we would be there for their birth, we would be. Women talked to each other, and the word of mouth recommendation was important. Women said that they had been let down many times: by family, partners and services. We tried to be very clear about what we could and could not do. Occasionally, officers would not call us for a birth, and it would feel terrible to have let a woman down, but women generally understood that this was out of our control. We had to say to women that we would do our very best to be with them at birth but that we could not guarantee this.

Birth Companions learned how important it was to be reliable and trustworthy. Many things were not within our power, and sometimes we could only listen. Nevertheless, listening could be very powerful. Birth companions would sometimes come away from a prison visit feeling bad that they had not made any difference. A couple of weeks later, a woman would tell us how much "lighter" she had felt that day after she was listened to.

13.4   How Services Developed

It has always been important for Birth Companions to ask women what they thought about our services. We learned a lot from what women said and also from the evaluation forms that we asked women to complete. This confirmed that our approach felt right but also told us what else women needed, and we tried to develop our services to meet these needs. Women told us that there were many barriers to breastfeeding in prison, and we developed a specific role and group around breastfeeding support. This led to breastfeeding rates that were actually higher than those in the community* (add footnote). However, women who were bottle feeding felt left out, so we included all the mothers on the Mother and Baby Unit and changed the name of the group to "early parenting". Women in prison are entitled to equivalence of healthcare to women in the community, but women told us of many instances when this care was compromised by being in prison, and we began work on a Birth Charter for women in prison, with 15 recommendations for improving care (link to Birth Charter). We worked with women to write the Birth Charter so that they could have a voice, and it included many direct quotes [8].

Women also told us that, sometimes, after being released, they would have less support and would be giving birth alone; they wished our support could continue. Therefore, we developed a Community Link service in London to support women post-release. We also decided to accept referrals from the Helen Bamber Foundation for women who had been trafficked. These women had experienced trauma and were also separated from family and community and giving birth with little or no support. Like the women in prison, they faced many challenges, and we adopted a similar approach: building trust, creating safety and listening.

As Birth Companions has developed, we have been able to offer women in the community different options and services in London. Pregnant women can come to our targeted antenatal classes, which are designed to make women feel safe and included. The course content and class facilitators do not assume that a woman has a partner, is in good housing or will be able to stay with her baby after the birth. We also have a Mother and Baby group which meets weekly, and women can start to attend in pregnancy. There is birth support and one-to-one visits. We understand that women's situations are different and that they have different needs and will make different choices. Some women find coming to a group difficult and opt instead for a 1:1 support. The fact that a woman is marginalised and facing challenges in her life may mean that she has become disempowered, but it does not mean that she should not be offered something that is tailored to her needs. Assumptions are often made about women from particular backgrounds or who are facing challenges in their lives so that they are given less choice or information. We offer a woman some options and let her decide what will be best for her. Choice and empowerment are important.

13.5   The Essence of How We Work

A few years ago, we came together as staff, sessional workers and volunteers to think about all the different elements of our approach and to describe our way of working. Words like "non-judgemental", "unconditional", "woman-centred", "kind", "reliable", "confidential" and "safe" kept coming up. Women often tell us that we are different from the other organisations and people who they meet, and we thought about all the feedback that women have given us. They like that we do not ask them too many questions and that they do not have to keep explaining their situation in order to qualify for our support. They like that we listen instead of telling them what to do.

Women in the community, like the women in prison, also tell us that they do not want to feel defined by the difficulties that they are facing and that they want to feel like a "normal" pregnant woman or mum. One woman who we supported at birth wrote:

> My pregnancy was really traumatic- I did worry that I would have problems as a mum, but the positive birth experience helped me so much. Birth Companions are the most accepting and understanding group of women I have ever met. There was no judgement, they never made me feel like the reason they were there was because I was a vulnerable mother .... I get a lot of help from services and I really appreciate that people are really kind to me but I'm always aware that those services are there because of my experiences. With Birth Companions there was none of that. There was nothing that made me feel different from any other mother which I think is so important for vulnerable women. (Katelyn)

Women have good reasons for asking for our support, so we will support a woman for her birth even if she has a partner or family around her. Sometimes, women have undergone experiences that are too painful or difficult to share with their family, or sometimes, the family have also experienced violence or trauma, and the woman knows that supporting her at her birth may be triggering for them. Although women are in very challenging situations, they often have great insight into what will be difficult for them and what sort of support they will need, so we try to be flexible. One woman told us that she felt extremely anxious and could only come to our antenatal classes if we met her at home and came with her to the first one. We did this, and then she was able to attend on her own.

13.6   A Trauma-Informed Approach

After working for many years, we realised that our approach was what was coming to be known as a "trauma-informed approach" and that there was a body of litera-ture about this [9, 10]. Although we did not deliver a service specifically about trauma, the understanding that any woman we met may have experienced trauma informed the way that we worked. One of our volunteers, who is also a midwife, compared this to the way a midwife will put on gloves for all women as part of "universal precautions". We attended workshops run by Stephanie Covington, who had developed a programme around trauma for women in prison in the USA. Stephanie advocates the need for gender-specific services because the experi-ences and impact of trauma on women and men are very different. Women are far more likely to experience violence and trauma in their interpersonal relationships; for men, it is more likely to be from a stranger or external source such as war. She refers to the five key elements (identified by Harris and Fallot (2001) *Using Trauma Theory to Design Service Systems*) [11] for providing a trauma-informed service for women which are safety, trustworthiness, choice, collaboration and empowerment. It has been very helpful for Birth Companions to have this more theoretical under-standing of our approach and why it works.

Stephanie Covington and others have written about how to create a feeling of safety for women coming into an office or centre [12]. Some spaces are full of posters or signs that can evoke feelings of alarm and distress, however well inten-tioned: posters about violence and abuse, warnings that violence against staff will not be tolerated, signs listing items or behaviour that are not allowed or uncom-fortable furniture and areas that are open and do not allow confidentiality. A com-pletely different atmosphere can be created by using posters with soothing images, welcome signs, flowers, comfortable furniture, refreshments and confidential spaces. Many women's centres have adopted this approach, and Trevi House (http://www.trevihouse.org) [13] is a good example of a centre that has been using a trauma-informed approach for a number of years. Stephanie also advocates that centres and organisations do a regular "walk through" of their services through the eyes of a woman: her first contact and then her journey through the service.

Some clinic and hospital waiting areas have been really improved by using the "walk through" and trauma-informed "make-over" of spaces, at a very minimal cost.

Birth Companions has worked for over 20 years without having an office or space to meet women in, so safety has to be conveyed in other ways. In prison, we welcome women into a room that is nevertheless a prison space, but we greet women, do introductions, are respectful, listen and provide refreshments. The groups are not compulsory, so it is the woman's choice to attend, and we talk about consent and the choices women can make. Women often say that they are understanding for the first time that an internal examination requires her consent. Many have had previous births, and either have not been asked for their consent or were asked in such a way that they did not realise that declining was an option. The groups provide women with evidence-based information so that they can make choices. In these various ways, we try to create a space that is empowering and conducive to wellbeing. Recently, one of the prisons decided to make our group compulsory, and this changed the dynamic dramatically. Some women became resentful and told us they did not want to be there.

In the community, we offer to go to a woman's home to meet her, so she can be in a relaxed space; but this is not always the case. A woman may be on a friend's sofa or living in a hostel dorm and not have privacy. Some women are living with abusive partners. If meeting at home does not feel good for a woman, we ask where she would like to meet. This could be in a café or at the antenatal clinic. We try to respect her wishes and create a feeling of trust wherever we are meeting, much as we do in the group. Even in the first communication with a woman, by phone or text, we want to let her know that we are trauma-informed: through our tone of voice, language and honouring her concerns. We have noticed that a significant number of women who have requested birth support actually go into labour soon after first meeting with us. It is as if they feel reassured that they will not be on their own and can then allow labour to happen. The importance of conveying safety and reassurance and the capacity to do this, even in the most adverse conditions, are described very powerfully by a former staff member, who is also a psychotherapist. She wrote about her interactions, in her Birth Companions role, with women not able to attend our groups (women may have had other visits or classes or felt too fragile to do so):

> Some of the women we visited away from the group setting would be in shared cells. Sometimes it wasn't possible for an officer to unlock the women. When we saw women in this circumstance, we would talk to her through the hatch of her cell door. The hatch is a small window with a flap, big enough to see the middle third of someone's face when up close. I spent many hours supporting women in this scenario. Talking and listening through the hatch… The women were often distressed. Some had just arrived, just separated from a baby they had to leave at court or at home. Some had been breastfeeding until very recently and were trying to manage the pain of both separation and engorged breasts. Some were pregnant and getting to grips with the realisation that their baby may be born while they are serving a prison sentence. These were highly emotional and difficult interactions. These women desperately needed to talk and to be listened to, and all of

this happened through a hatch, with me, a woman they had never met before. There would often be other women in the cell behind her talking or watching TV, and a lot of activity in the corridor behind me, officers escorting prisoners, doors and gates opening and closing. For that time she and I worked hard at make the most of the time we had together. It was my intention to support the woman and show compassion and kindness in this less than perfect environment. I attempted to use my knowledge and therapeutic skills to develop a short-term relationship with the woman, in a way that would be helpful to her. Through regularly being in this position I have learnt a great deal. Before I had worked in this way, I thought that it would be useless to spend a short amount of time with someone in a noisy setting with a physical door between you both. Since the experience I have learned that quite the opposite to be true. Although far from ideal, it is possible to develop a good enough relationship and provide support to someone in distress with all of the limitations of the prison environment. Women have said that the contact made a positive difference to their wellbeing, which has been a great eye opener and reminder to me of the power of kindness, compassion and unconditional support whatever the restrictions of the environment .... [14]

13.7 Woman-to-Woman Peer Support

Birth Companions began as woman-to-woman peer support, offered by a small group of volunteers to women giving birth from Holloway prison. Although Birth Companions now has 9 part-time staff, and over 30 active sessional workers and volunteers, the support model is similar. We have paid Co-ordinators for the projects and a mixture of volunteers and sessional workers delivering the groups and one-to-one support, but all birth support is done on a voluntary basis. This volunteer element seems to be important, and health professionals and prison officers often remark on it, that someone has come out in the middle of the night to be at a birth and isn't being paid. The women we work with are less aware of who is paid and who is not but often comment on the special nature of the support.

There is definitely something about creating a sense of community and inclusion for women who are feeling isolated and on the margins of society. One woman who we supported at birth and was due to be separated from her baby later wrote "At first I did not think they would be able to help someone like me…" Another said: "I had no family or friends by my side during pregnancy and birth, but I wasn't alone-Birth Companions became my family". One of our volunteers described our birth support in the community in London as being like:

a moveable village or family- a network of brilliant women ready to assemble … at almost a moment's notice to ensure that these most precious moments (for mums and babies) *… are as they should be- surrounded and supported by women.* (Volunteer)

Another type of peer support happens in our groups. We first noticed this in the prison groups, where more established women would support the newer women who had just come into prison, explaining how the system worked and also giving reassurance. This also happens, in different ways, in our community groups. We realise that by providing the safe spaces and modelling inclusive behaviour, we are enabling women to support each other.

13.8 Participation and Collaboration

A few years ago, we carried out a research project with women who we had supported in the community a couple of years earlier. Although women had said this
before, we were surprised at how many women said that they wanted to give something back, help other women and stay involved with Birth Companions. More
recently, some generous funding has enabled us to do this. We have trained former
service users as peer supporters and peer researchers and provided volunteering
opportunities both inside and outside Birth Companions. For many years, we have
invited women who wanted to stay in touch to a lunch and discussion day once or
twice a year. Women told us that in order to be able to attend, meetings needed to be
on a Saturday and that a crèche was essential. Also, some women requested that the
crèche be in a separate room so that they could speak more openly. This was particularly an issue for women who had been in prison but also for women who had been
trafficked and had experiences that they did not want their children to overhear.
Women really value these opportunities to get together and share experiences, as
well as having the chance to give their views and feedback and stay connected with
Birth Companions. For the women who had been in prison, these get-togethers
seemed to be particularly powerful; some told us that it had been the first time that
they had felt able to talk about their prison experiences since being released 2, 3 or
even 4 years earlier. We realised, yet again, the importance of the trust that had been
built and of providing a "safe space". The recent funding has enabled us to develop
a Lived Experience Team (LET) so that women who wanted to support the work of
Birth Companions and stay involved can now meet quarterly, still on a Saturday and
with a crèche.

13.9 Looking After Staff and Volunteers

The first birth companions had extensive birth support experience, but as the organisation grew, we developed a training programme which enabled us to recruit more
widely. We accepted volunteers who brought many skills and insights, were highly
motivated to support women and may have had their own perinatal experience, but
had not necessarily worked in this area before. Our training now includes 8 core
days and covers boundaries, lone working, self-care and safeguarding, as well as
perinatal topics. Although our approach is warm and caring, and women often say
that the birth companions are like friends or family, the volunteers are trained to
support women in a way that is safe and professional. This protects the women and
the volunteers.

In the community, a staff member meets all women initially and co-ordinates the
support. We try to have two to three volunteers involved with each woman, so she is
clear that the relationship is with Birth Companions rather than with a particular
volunteer. Volunteers sometimes need to take a break, because of other commitments, and we do not want women to feel let down. It can also sometimes feel
overwhelming for a volunteer to feel she is the only person in a woman's life, and

we do not want to create a feeling of dependence for women. If a volunteer is not clear about the relationship, this can be confusing for women, so we give volunteers a code of practice and support to work within this. Volunteers are asked not to share their personal numbers or maintain the relationship once the support has come to an end. This is different from the way most doulas work and was hard for some volunteers. However, we have learned that if volunteers are going to be able to continue and not become overwhelmed, they do need this distance. For the woman, although we are supporting her and her baby through an incredibly important time, we are wanting to empower her to find her own strength and to start to build her own support network for the future.

We have realised that the trauma-informed approach is important, not only for the women we support but also for our volunteers, staff and sessional workers. Without looking after these people, the work of Birth Companions is not sustainable. The original group of volunteers supported each other with the difficult situations that they were encountering in the prison. They met monthly in a comfortable space, with refreshments, to talk about the births, and they also debriefed in between meetings, one to one on the phone or by meeting up.

Today we use a similar model across our various projects, although the numbers of people involved have now increased five- or sixfold. Each project has a small team with a Co-ordinator who can debrief with volunteers and sessional staff after visits, groups and supporting women at birth. There are regular team meetings over a nice lunch or in the evening with snacks. People need to feel nurtured and food is important. This is true of our staff and volunteers, as well as the women in our prison and community groups. We hold regular training, to continue our learning and development, and socials, so everyone in the organisation can relax and get to know each other. We ask our volunteers for feedback: what they value in Birth Companions and what could be better. On the whole, volunteers feel well supported and valued. In fact, many tell us that the same level of support has not existed for them in other organisations. At other times, when there has been a particularly difficult birth or situation, volunteers have told us that they needed more support, and we responded. We held additional meetings so that all those who had been involved in the difficult birth or situation could come together and debrief as a group.

Our awareness about vicarious traumatisation has increased, and we talk more about this in our trainings and meetings. Five years ago, we introduced a training about recognising stress and using relaxation techniques. A couple of years ago, we trialled a Reflective Practice group for volunteers run by a group therapist. A couple of volunteers really benefitted, but most could not fit this additional support into their already busy lives; others told us they already felt well supported. We began a similar monthly session for staff (in addition to a monthly supervision that all staff have with their line manager). Most staff have direct contact with the women we are supporting and see them for the initial meeting and/or are main facilitators of the prison and community groups. They are dealing with very difficult stories and situations. As one staff member said:

At one point I realised that the women in the (prison) *group were separated from 16 babies or children. I felt the enormity of their grief. I had to share this feeling with someone and talked about it in my Reflective Practice session.* (Birth Companion staff member)

This additional therapeutic support is proving beneficial for staff and will, hopefully, also better enable staff to support the sessional workers and volunteers in their teams.

13.10 Challenges

Although being "trauma-informed" is firmly embedded in the way that we work with women, it is harder to keep hold of this approach when it comes to looking after ourselves. The temptation for staff and volunteers can be to give too much of themselves, and this can impact on wellbeing and family life. We have always encouraged volunteers to take a break when going through demanding or difficult times. It is hard to support others unless you are feeling well resourced yourself. We are continuing to learn and, this year, have run two training sessions about trauma, both with a strong self-care element, attended by over 30 staff and volunteers.

We have also learned that change needs to be managed carefully. When we first started to support women in the community many years ago, some experienced volunteers felt overwhelmed, and we had not anticipated this. We assumed that supporting women in the community would be easier than in prison, but in prison there are many boundaries. We see women within a set time period and place and are only allowed to give women certain items (such as bras for breastfeeding). When we leave after a prison visit, we know that a woman will have someone to talk to and basic food and shelter. In the community, our volunteers found it harder to come away from a visit, knowing that a woman was completely alone. Some women we supported in hospital could not go back to their hostel with their baby and were homeless after giving birth. We realised that community support brought new challenges, and we developed a training and guidelines specifically for this work.

We would like to be able to support more women but do not want to lose what the women, and also our volunteers, like about us. If we continued to expand, we would struggle to find funding. Increasingly, we are trying to improve conditions by doing influencing work and by giving the women we work with a voice: through speaking at conferences, writing articles and carrying out research. We are speaking more to decision-makers, prisons, health professionals and others working with perinatal women about the challenges faced by women with complex needs and the need for a trauma-informed approach.

13.11 Conclusion

Unfortunately, women with complex needs continue to have negative experiences of services. Women tell us about having to retell their story several times within the same organisation, about feeling judged, about having to answer personal and upsetting questions in a space without privacy, about going to a group where no one spoke to them, about not being clear about what would happen next and about not feeling safe and not being listened to. Listening to these experiences, it is hard not to conclude that it is the services, rather than the women, that can be "difficult to engage with".

Our experience in Birth Companions has been that women with complex needs can be highly motivated to engage with a service in the perinatal period, as long as this feels safe and beneficial for a woman and her baby. We have seen this positive engagement with specialist midwifery teams and other services, as well as with Birth Companions. Although experiences of trauma and having been let down can make women more wary of services, there is much that can be done through adopting a trauma-informed approach.

References

1. Marshall D. Birth companions: working with women in prison giving birth. Br J Midwifery. 2010;18(4):225–8.
2. Beech BAL. Birth in chains. AIMS J. 1996;7(4):4–6.
3. Worley E. Gentle birth companions-doulas serving humanity. Midwives. 2011;14(7):44.
4. https://hibiscusinitiatives.org.uk/
5. Bennett R. Maternity care reform in English prisons: a century of unanswered concerns. History & Policy; 2019.
6. Simkin P. Birth partner: a complete guide to childbirth for dads, partners, doulas, and all other labor companions. 5th ed. Beverly, USA: Harvard Common Press; 2018.
7. Simkin P, Klaus P. When survivors give birth. Seattle, WA: Classic Day; 2004.
8. Kennedy A, Marshall D, Parkinson D, Delap N, Abbott L. Birth charter for women in prisons in England and Wales. London, UK: Birth Companions; 2016.
9. Covington SS, Burke C, Keaton S, Norcott C. Evaluation of a trauma-informed and gender-responsive intervention for women in drug treatment. J Psychoactive Drugs. 2008;40(Suppl 5):387–98.
10. Sperlich M, Seng JS, Li Y, Taylor J, Bradbury-Jones C. Integrating trauma-informed care into maternity care practice: conceptual and practical issues. J Midwifery Womens Health. 2017;62(6):661–72.
11. Harris ME, Fallot RD. Using trauma theory to design service systems. New York: Jossey-Bass; 2001.
12. Covington SS, Bloom BE. Gender responsive treatment and services in correctional settings. Women Ther. 2007;29(3-4):9–33.
13. Shead H. ONE-TO-ONE. Midwives. 2015;18(1):19.
14. Credit: Previous Birth Companions staff member: Katie Bottle.

Conclusion

14

Laura Abbott

Pursuing a multidisciplinary approach, our book represented a joined-up style of best practice discussions in relation to pregnant women and new mothers who may have complex needs. Our book brought together a blend of healthcare professionals, people with lived experiences and charity experts with proficiency in caring for and supporting perinatal women with complex social issues. We reiterated the necessity of meeting the needs of women who may face complex issues and how we may achieve this. An overarching aim has been to find ways to deliver multi-agency continuity of care, whilst being aware of bias, professional responsibilities and an understanding how we can take a holistic approach—essential for attaining excellence in twenty-first-century maternity care provision. We hope that through the knowledge gained includes the importance of third sector partnerships, working in tandem with women who are experts by experiences and bringing health professionals together.

Each chapter invited the reader to step into the shoes of the perinatal woman. The latest Mothers and Babies: Reducing Risk through Audits and Confidential Enquiries across the UK (MBRRACE-UK) [1] blatantly demonstrates the consequences that having multiple complexities has and the need to ensure that susceptible groups receive personalised, appropriate care. Through our collective writing, we provided a paradigm for partnership working and hope to have strengthened voices by highlighting diverse experiences. In combination with recommendations from specialists in the field, we have offered a unique mix of compassion and evidence-based guidance, addressing a range of social issues, and provided essential information. We have looked at how using a trauma-informed approach can be applied universally to care for all women. We have read about and heard from charities such as

L. Abbott (✉)

Department of Allied Health and Midwifery, University of Hertfordshire, Hatfield, Hertfordshire, UK

e-mail: l.abbott@herts.ac.uk

Birth Companions, the 4M Project and the Salamander Trust how different approaches may directly impact women's care in a positive and holistic way.

In *Naomi Delap's* opening chapter (Chap. 2), the reader was introduced to the concept of embedding trauma-informed approaches into our practice. Adverse Childhood Experiences (ACEs) were explored in relation to the impact upon the pregnant woman. Drawing upon the pioneering work of Dr Stephanie Covington, Delap explained how a universal and targeted style of adopting a trauma-informed approach to care is one that maternity services should implement. Delap detailed:

> *"Pregnancy and childbirth is a period which survivors of the trauma of childhood and adult sexual abuse may find particularly challenging; in which the potential for women to be re-traumatised is significant".*

Delap draws from current studies that demonstrate that women with extensive experience of physical and sexual violence will be far more likely to experience disadvantage and inequality in other areas of their lives, including poverty and debt, poor living conditions, physical and mental ill health and disability, substance dependence, homelessness and discrimination. These experiences of extreme trauma, particularly those that start during childhood, have an adverse impact on women's lives. Delap infers that most of the women who have experienced extensive physical and sexual violence as children and who go on to have children will pass through maternity services, with a significant number of women giving birth doing so with a background of trauma.

The partnership model philosophy the charity Birth Companions that Delap directs was identified as especially important. Working collaboratively with women demonstrates how women with lived experiences inform their guidance and care. This model of working runs as a golden thread through our book. Angelina Namiba, Longret Kwardem, Rebecca Mbewe, Fungai Murau, Susan Bewley, Shema Tariq and Alice Welbourn demonstrate this in their Chap. 10 describing the 4M Programme, a perinatal peer mentoring project led by, with and for women living with HIV in the UK. Working alongside and with women who have lived experience is also described by Denise Marshall MBE (Chap. 13) and Abbi Ayers (Chap. 12). On describing what a trauma-informed maternity services will look like, Delap emphasised the need to include the women our services are designed for, every step of the way.

Jennifer Parker's Chap. 5 examined perinatal mental health, looking specifically at the experience of women undergoing IVF and the potential for antenatal anxiety and perinatal mental health. Current research and literature were explored in relation to current practices in maternity and whether they are enough to support the perinatal woman with antenatal anxiety. Recommendations for practice were made to include further enhancement in midwifery education in perinatal mental health. Linking a common theme running through our book—the underlying stigma caused by having mental ill health was discussed:

> Less than half of those living with mental health illness seek treatment and stigma is the most significant impediment to seeking mental healthcare. Mental health is stigmatised at three levels: self, social/public and structural. These levels interact with one another,

mutually reinforcing the associated stigma. When people with mental illness believe preju-
dices and discredited stereotypes regarding those with mental illness, this leads to
self-stigma.

Parker relayed the importance of the midwife's role and responsibility in assessing signs of normal or worsening mental health. Midwives can have a positive impact, especially when adopting continuity of care models delivered with a holistic, collaborative and woman-centred approach.

Suzanne Reynolds' Chap. 6 about homelessness in the pregnant population applied her innovative qualitative research alongside experience as a specialist midwife for homeless women to highlight the impact of women's experience entering homelessness during pregnancy. Research surrounding the experiences and impact of women experiencing homelessness during pregnancy is limited, yet the impact of an out-of-home situation on the mother and developing child is far-reaching, affecting physical, mental and emotional wellbeing. Reynolds illuminates the experiences of women enduring homelessness and draws us to consider the umbrella term of homelessness. This considers not only women residing in hostels or experiencing street homelessness but those living in insecure or inadequate accommodation. Conceptualising homelessness in this way, Reynolds offered a more inclusive and nuanced approach, highlighting that homelessness is not limited to people living rough but having an impact far more detrimental than simply requiring a "roof over one's head". Reynolds reflects on why there is such limited guidance for midwives and maternity services and how we should adapt maternity services to support pregnant women experiencing homelessness, summarised in the overall themes of her research:

> *Women recounted feelings of imprisonment within their rooms due to the location and*
> *inflexible rules of the emergency accommodation, leading to their social isolation when*
> *they were feeling most vulnerable. They also cited a lack of solicitude towards them from*
> *frontline workers, inadequate and poorly located accommodation and an absence of dedi-*
> *cated services as challenging their perceptions of pregnancy being a "priority need" and*
> *led women to push aside their pregnancy and not be "present" to focus on their develop-*
> *ing baby.*

Reynolds submits that there is a growing body of evidence that supports the harmful consequences of homelessness on families, yet there is a scarcity of literature describing the experiences or journey of a pregnant women into homelessness. Themes such as instability, stress and lack of control are common with women commenting on the high levels of distress, mental health issues, isolation and lack of social support they experience upon becoming homeless. This chapter explored the legal frameworks and social issues that influence the pathway that the pregnant woman may take through homelessness, the effect an out-of-home situation has on the pregnancy, birth outcomes and child development and offered recommendations for good clinical practice within maternity services.

Karen Mills' Chap. 4 on substance misuse considered the relationship between substance misuse and risk in parenting with this triangulation of risk, need and strength in women who are or are about to become parents. Links with trauma experienced by a person addicted to drugs as a form of self-medication are understandable, especially when we examine the experiences outlined in Chaps. 2, 8, 12, and 13 by Delap, Marshall, Ayers and Abbott. Used to alter mood and perception, drugs are widely available in UK society. They are consumed to alter bodily systems for a medical purpose and extend into social and recreational circumstances. Mills explained that "drug use" is a common phenomenon which includes aspirin and chocolate as well as alcohol and illegal drugs. Problematic drug use is somewhat different related to both health and social problems. A consequence of substance misuse is that it can become the leading focus of a person's life, potentially having a deleterious impact on parenting capacity. Chapter 4 draws upon evidence and reports to consider the benefits and pitfalls of multi-agency practice:

> They (parents) *may deny or understate their drug use or may act to avoid support services where substance misuse will be uncovered. Injuries and deaths to children have occurred repeatedly where workers have been overly influenced by the plausible rationale for events offered by the parent and not stepped back to make an assessment which is centred on the safety of the child.*

Mills drew specifically upon Serious Case Reviews to indicate areas where health and midwifery services need to be more cognisant of risk to children and infants and more able to bring their assessment of risk to safeguarding services. Mills identified that drug and alcohol use is implicated in a high percentage of serious case reviews with the complexity of a family's struggles rather than drug use per se which precipitates risk. These difficulties are often revealed as a combination of drug use with domestic violence (see Chap. 7) or mental ill health (see Chap. 5), often stemming from their own childhood trauma (see Chap. 2). Where this is the case, the risk to children is considerable with women also perceived as isolated, anxious as well as physically hurt. Mills recommends good multi-agency liaison, due to these risks, and with an understanding of the stigma surrounding these complexities.

Tawanda Bvumburai (Chap. 3) writes about the experiences of Black, Asian and Minority Ethnic women (BAME) in her Chap. 3. Bvumburai shines a light on the disparities that Black women may experience, especially in maternity care. Bvumburai outlines how the evolution of racism plays a key part on the inequalities and maps the history of racism and the perpetuation of cultural myths in the UK. The statistics shows that Black women and babies are at increased risk of dying in maternity, with Black women five times more likely to die and Asian women twice more likely to die than their white counterparts [1]. The incidences of deaths of babies that are born to Black, Asian and women in Minority Ethnic groups have the highest infant mortality rate in the UK. Bvumburai suggests that bias and racism are learnt rather than inherent which suggests that it can be unlearnt too. Therefore, responsibility lies with meaningful training and working with maternity services, campaign groups and the third sector to turn the tide against the shameful record of mortality and morbidity for the BAME community. Auditing Black and Asian women about their experiences of maternity care, Bvumburai asked about their experience alongside midwives' experiences of caring for Black, Asian and Minority Ethnic women. The snapshot of findings demonstrated a true reflection of what the statistics illustrate with a call for change and further research. Bvumburai identified that often the racism was not immediately obvious, but an undercurrent existed:

> *"I don't think I've outwardly witnessed racism, but I definitely feel a lack of effort in people's care towards BAME women. Especially when there's a language barrier involved."*

Bvumburai suggested that the beliefs outside of the healthcare environment influences the workplace and will be interlaced into everything and recommends a national drive forward with training and policies. The words of a Black woman who received care in the 1980s were particularly poignant:

> *"The Midwives would wash all the other babies and leave my baby and so I just got on with it and washed my baby myself. They would also take all the other babies to the nursery at night, so the mums could get sleep, but they would never take mine."*

This chapter explored the statistics, research and history involved in Black Asian and Ethnic minority women's experiences of maternity care. Of prominence was the history, lived experiences and professional recommendations of what can be done to tackle disparities. The impetus for positive change in response to the reports and responses from women were highlighted by Bvumburai, adding evidence to campaigns and inquiries such as FIVEXMORE and Birthrights [2, 3]. It was also written in the hope that it will evoke positive change and help consistently bring positive outcomes.

Celia Wildeman's Chap. 7 on Domestic violence and abuse in pregnancy enables midwives to become more aware of the key communication elements such as the verbal and non-verbal cues that women might exhibit, indicating the negative treatment they may endure. Wildeman has counselled women therapeutically for over 30 years and draws upon her knowledge and experience of the devastation that violence and abuse causes to family's lives. The chapter suggests language that best facilitates disclosure, trust and respect by providing examples of best midwifery practice. It also aims to encourage midwives to be more reflective in their own practice to enable learning and change to occur.

It is well-known that violence and abuse can occur at any time in a relationship, but for some women, it is initiated or escalated during pregnancy. Wildeman described how violence and abuse of pregnant and newly birthed women by an intimate partner is a complex issue because of the individual nature of its manifestation with potentially serious consequences for the woman, unborn baby and wider family. Wildeman examines the evidence that suggests that some midwives do not feel able to deal with the complexity of domestic abuse (DA) and domestic violence (DV). Indeed, as a mainly female workforce, midwives will undoubtedly be included in the statistics of women experiencing DV/DA themselves. With this in mind, it is important to link back to Delap's Chap. 2 of what a trauma-informed maternity service could look like and a trauma-informed health service in general. Wildeman found that sometimes midwives lacked confidence to ask questions about women's experiences of DV/DA. This would sometimes be due to the uncertainty of how they might manage confirmation:

"It could open a can of worms and what would I then do?"

Wildeman reported that students too felt that they had not received the training and guidance that would enable them to feel confident to question a woman's DV/DA history and be able to work in a confident and knowledgeable way. Wildeman recommended that policy frameworks and guidance reflect the evidence and that training programs are meaningful and tailored rather than a tick box exercise.

Laura Abbott's Chap. 8 discussed the evidence relating to pregnant women and new mothers in prison. It is understood that many women who end up in the criminal justice system are from extremely disadvantaged backgrounds. With similar themes arising around the complex backgrounds of women, this chapter, like Delap's, Ayer's and Marshall's, recommended adopting a universal trauma-informed approach. It is reported that a substantial percentage of women in prison are survivors of sexual abuse and neglect in childhood, may have been in the care of the local authority, may have been homeless and may be survivors of domestic violence. Often because of having endured trauma, women may use drugs and alcohol as a form of self-medication against emotional pain, as discussed in Chap. 4. In light of these histories, it is unsurprising that a high proportion of women in prison suffer from mental ill health and complex post-traumatic stress disorder [4].

Women in prison at particularly high risk of health complications in pregnancy and Abbott's Chap. 8 reflected the experience of pregnant women in prison, considering their maternity care needs for each trimester and during the post-natal period. The chapter gave an overview of the current research undertaken, in view of the demographics and characteristics of women who may become incarcerated, their health outcomes and the psychological impact of imprisonment. Vignettes illuminated the experiences of women in relation to human rights, toxic stress, the fear of going into labour at night, the shame experienced and the impact of being separated from their baby. Abbott asked the reader to contemplate being in the imprisoned woman's shoes through empathetic consideration:

Close your eyes. Imagine your perspective of what a prison looks like and how it might feel to be inside. Envisage the environment and what the atmosphere may feel like. Now imagine a pregnant woman in her last trimester. Place her in that environment. Consider how she may be feeling. What do you think her worries and concerns may be?

Throughout the chapter, the reader is asked to anticipate their professional responsibilities and, like other chapters, to look at their own potential misconceptions when caring for the pregnant prisoner. The author's own novel qualitative research further illuminates the experiences of pregnant women in prison and those being supported by charities such as Birth Companions, demonstrating the importance of care and compassion shown by third sector organisations.

Angelina ba, Longret Kwardem, Rebecca Mbewe, Fungai Murau, Susan Bewley, Shema Tariq and *Alice Welbourn's* Chap. 10 described the 4M Programme, a perinatal peer mentoring project led by, with and for women living with HIV in the UK. It considered HIV and pregnancy both within a UK and a global context, describing the epidemiology as well as policy and practice. The authors described the first UK grassroots charity-led Mentor Mother programme also led by, and for, women living with HIV. Hosted by Positively UK, Angelina Namiba, one of the chapter's co-authors, and a co-Director of 4M Mentor Mothers Network CIC, created the original programme. Describing the success of the programme, the authors stated:

> There is good evidence of the efficacy of perinatal peer support in improving psychosocial, health and behavioural outcomes in pregnancy. Specifically, in HIV, it has been shown to have positive psychosocial impacts, with improvements in clinical outcomes in randomised controlled trials.

The Chaps. 2, 12, and 13 demonstrated the importance of partnership working with women who are experts through experience, leading specifically to positive outcomes for women who live with HIV. Similar to Bvumburai's Chap. 3, racial stereotypes and their deep-rooted histories are discussed, especially in relation to the disproportionate criminalisation of Black, Indigenous and other women of colour for relatively minor transgressions, such as drug use in pregnancy:

> Childbirth with HIV is perhaps the most recent example of an enduring, unacceptable, societal prejudice towards women and babies deemed to exist outside the straitjacket of prevailing social norms.

The programme linked Mentor Mothers to healthcare providers and HIV charities and trained women living with HIV as Mentor Mothers, so that each could work as part of a multidisciplinary team of health- and social care providers to support women living with HIV throughout their pregnancies. Each Mentor Mother was also linked to a local HIV charity, to receive ongoing support. The programme ran successfully from 2010 to 2015, when funding ceased. A formal evaluation demonstrated positive multidimensional impacts on women's emotional wellbeing whilst leading to personal growth among Mentor Mothers themselves. This co-written, co-produced chapter models the equal partnership working between experts by experience and professionals.

Paulina Sporek de Lacerda's Chap. 11 illuminated the experiences of maternity services for deaf women. The chapter discussed the limited research into experiences of deaf women in the perinatal period. Sporek de Lacerda founded the Deaf Nest Project with the aim to improve pregnant Deaf users' personal experience, equality of access and choice and control over maternity care. The chapter highlighted the need to train midwives and other healthcare professionals in becoming deaf aware with the associated communication skills. The lack of relevant literature suggested that deafness and pregnancy are two concepts rarely considered together. Despite the most recently available statistic which shows a dramatic increase in hearing loss, little has been said or done in relation to pregnancy and childbirth. Those barriers limit women's psycho-emotional wellbeing with links between social exclusion, vulnerability and adverse pregnancy outcomes (MBRRACE-UK) [1]. Deaf parents may face considerable obstacles in their journey of parenthood:

> *After having my baby, I was on the ward and my buzzer didn't work, and I was told that the midwives were aware of my hearing loss as I was worried I wouldn't be able to hear my baby cry at night. But they didn't let me know when she was crying, I just simply didn't sleep for 24 hours! I do feel frustrated that deaf parents are not given accessible information. I would like to think that I have a support network around me available like hearing people have.*

Pregnancy and motherhood are major life events for all women, not least for Deaf women. Nevertheless, they need to be accepted and supported in their choice to become parents and to be cared for and treated like every other woman. Sporek de Lacerda discussed the role of midwife throughout pregnancy and the post-natal period starting with the first booking appointment. The chapter introduced us to information about the medical versus cultural models and includes useful information regarding British sign Language and lip reading. Myths and misconceptions about the Deaf community are discussed, alongside the common thread running through our book—stigma. Sporek de Lacerda states that the Deaf population are commonly educated below their capacity, employed below their capability and viewed negatively by the hearing world.

Abbi Ayers's Chap. 12 discussed breastfeeding issues and challenges when a woman comes from a background of extreme disadvantage and complex social issues. Taking a trauma-informed approach, Ayers explored the key considerations health professionals, carers, policymakers and commissioners should adopt to ensure a trauma-informed breastfeeding support service for women with complex social needs. Current evidence and good practice demonstrated that when women with complex social needs accessed specialised breastfeeding support, the associated health and wellbeing outcomes improved. Ayers stated that:

> *The improved maternal, neonatal and long-term health and wellbeing benefits* (of breastfeeding) *are widely recognised and undisputed. However, the lesser understood and documented value that the breastfeeding experience holds for a mother recovering from trauma, abuse, poor mental health and multiple disadvantage is, at best, woefully under-estimated, and at worst, completely undermined by standard practice.*

Ayers described how breastfeeding support for women with complex social needs requires a proactive approach to understanding the barriers, triggers and inequalities they face when considering their infant feeding options. A proactive response is required to guarantee trauma-informed support that acknowledges and accounts for the multiple disadvantage, lived experience and deep-rooted trauma these women may bear. Like Delap's Chap. 2 explained, trauma-informed breastfeeding support would also work from the presumption that all women may have experienced or may currently be experiencing some form of trauma that might influence their infant feeding choices and compromise their natural ability to initiate and maintain breastfeeding:

> *If a clear grasp of the key principles of trauma-informed care remains at the centre of all our work with women with complex social needs, a trauma-informed model of breastfeeding support will evolve naturally.*

Ayers suggested that adopting a trauma-informed approach to breastfeeding support need not be complicated for health professionals and caregivers and that breastfeeding can offer health, hope and healing to women with complex social needs.

Denise Marshall MBE's Chap. 13 charted the history of the charity Birth Companions which began in 1996 after publicity about a woman from Holloway Prison being shackled in labour. The approach taken by the charity links to Delap and Ayer's Chaps. 2 and 12 in relation to trauma-informed methods as well as Abbott's Chap. 8 on the experiences of pregnant women in prison. The chapter explored the unique way that Birth Companions' work with women in prison and the community. The focus on listening to women is clearly outlined by Marshall who detailed that:

> *An aspect of the support was listening to women but not asking them about their offence or why they were in prison.*

The importance of working with women is illustrated in some of the feedback provided. An example of this is demonstrated in the quote below about how much women in prison felt valued as pregnant woman or a new mum, not a prisoner:

> "*When I arrived at the group, I felt so welcome, reassured and, even more importantly, accepted. I was encouraged to speak, never asked about why I was in prison and felt comfortable enough to open up about my hopes, fears and expectations as a mother to be. For two hours it felt like we were a normal group of mums and I can honestly say you forget where you are.*"

A key philosophy of Birth Companions was being non-judgemental and there to listen and support them as pregnant women, regardless of their history or why they were in prison. The severe environment of this early prison setting was a strong influence in shaping the ethos and way of working which now extends to working with women in the community who experience extreme disadvantage. Further, working in a trauma-informed way enlightens how the charity supports its own staff and volunteers—an ethos that Delap recommends in her Chap. 2 when discussing how a trauma-informed maternity service should look. Marshall provides useful insights for others working with women with complex needs in the perinatal period, both in the statutory and voluntary sectors.

Our book aimed to seek to increase our knowledge of some of the complexities facing women and their families. The chapters are written by experts in their field from a variety of backgrounds—either through experience, significant third sector expertise and bringing together their skills of peer care provision and an understanding of the unique needs of the women and families they support. It is the first piece of work to bring together a blend of healthcare professionals, people with lived experiences and charities with expertise in caring for and supporting perinatal women with complex social issues.

By highlighting experiences, voices have been amplified in our eclectic book. These are in turn combined with recommendations from specialists in the field, offering a unique mix of compassion, trauma-informed approaches and evidence-based guidance. It addressed a range of social issues and provided essential information and points for reflection and debate. This book will benefit all health- and social care professionals working in women's health whilst also providing a valuable reference guide for maternity departments. Blended working with women who are experts by experience, our third sector colleagues have demonstrated how we can balance giving the best quality care ensuring the woman's needs are always fundamental. Ultimately, we aim to culminate in a maternity service that delivers compassionate care to all women experiencing complex social needs and multiple disadvantage in a trauma-informed way.

References

1. Knight M, Bunch K, Tuffnell D, Shakespeare J, Kotnis R, Kenyon S, Kurinczuk JJ, editors. On behalf of MBRRACE-UK. Saving lives, improving mothers' care–lessons learned to inform maternity care from the UK and Ireland confidential enquiries into maternal deaths and morbidity 2016–18. Oxford: National Perinatal Epidemiology Unit, University of Oxford; 2020.
2. https://www.birthrights.org.uk/2021/02/07/new-inquiry-to-drive-action-on-racial-injustice-in-maternity-care/
3. https://www.fivexmore.com/
4. Corston J. The Corston report: a report by Baroness Jean Corston of a review of women with particular vulnerabilities in the criminal justice system: the need for a distinct, radically different, visibly-led, strategic, proportionate, holistic, woman centred, integrated approach. Home Office; 2007.

Printed in the United States
by Baker & Taylor Publisher Services